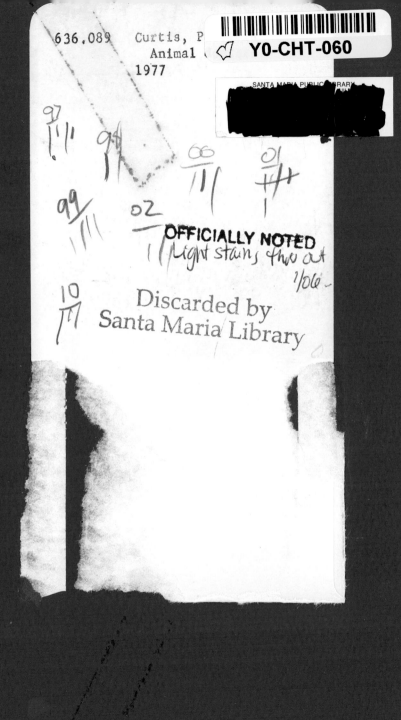

ANIMAL DOCTORS

ANIMAL DOCTORS

What It's Like to Be a Veterinarian
and How to Become One

Illustrated with photographs

PATRICIA CURTIS

DELACORTE PRESS / NEW YORK

Acknowledgments

From "Dolphins" by Brewster Ghiselin. Copyright © 1973 by The Modern Poetry Association; reprinted by permission of Brewster Ghiselin and *Poetry*. First published in *Poetry*, March 1973.

From "The Pasture" by Robert Frost. From *The Poetry of Robert Frost*, edited by Edward Connery Lathem. Copyright 1939, © 1967, 1969 by Holt, Rinehart and Winston. Reprinted by permission of Holt, Rinehart and Winston, Publishers.

Mark Twain quote used by permission of Harper & Row, Publishers, Inc.

Copyright © 1977 by Patricia Curtis

5-77 BT 195

Manufactured in the United States of America

First printing

Library of Congress Cataloging in Publication Data

Curtis, Patricia.
Animal doctors.

SUMMARY: Veterinarians discuss their attitudes toward their profession and describe their personal experiences. Supplementary information provides career guidance.
1. Veterinary medicine—Vocational guidance—Juvenile literature. 2. Veterinarians—Juvenile literature. [1. Veterinarians. 2. Veterinary medicine—Vocational guidance. 3. Vocational guidance] I. Title.

SF779.5.C87   636.089′069   76-5593

ISBN 0-440-00140-4

Contents

Photographs follow page 90.

Acknowledgments

With one exception (Dr. Henderson, the circus vet), all the veterinarians in these chapters are fictional characters, based loosely on real people. Some are composites of several people. But most of the stories come from real episodes in the lives of working veterinarians. Altogether, the comments and experiences of nineteen doctors of veterinary medicine provided me with my material.

I owe a special debt to Gary R. Bolton, DVM, for serving as my consultant in the preparation of this book. Dr. Bolton is Associate Professor of Cardiology in the Department of Small Animal Medicine and Surgery at New York State College of Veterinary Medicine, Cornell University. To be sure medical information in my chapters was accurate, I asked Dr. Bolton to read my manuscript and correct my mistakes. I was fortunate indeed to have his careful attention, his many corrections and suggestions, and his reassuring encouragement.

I also wish to thank the following veterinarians who were kind enough to allow me to interview them: Dr. John

Bandes of the Southbury Veterinary Hospital, Southbury, Connecticut; Dr. Robin Bandes of the Cheshire Veterinary Hospital, Cheshire, Connecticut; Dr. Emil P. Dolensek of the New York Zoological Park (Bronx Zoo); Dr. Ferris G. Gorra of Marble Dale, Connecticut; Dr. William D. Hardy, Jr. of the Memorial Sloan-Kettering Cancer Center, New York; Dr. J. Y. Henderson of Ringling Bros. Barnum & Bailey Circus; Dr. Lois E. Hinson, Dr. E. C. Sharman, and Dr. William R. Strieber of the Veterinary Services Division, Animal and Plant Health Inspection Service, U. S. Department of Agriculture; Dr. Jay D. Hyman of the Westchester Animal Hospital, Mt. Vernon, New York; Dr. Stephen C. Jaffe of Charlotte, North Carolina; Dr. Terri McGinnis of the Albany Veterinary Clinic, Albany, California; Dr. James L. Naviaux of Pleasant Hill, California; Dr. Jon Padover and Dr. Nancy Padover of the Morristown Animal Hospital, Morristown, New Jersey; Dr. James A. Pringle of the Westfield Animal Hospital, Pennsauken, New Jersey; Dr. Andre M. Ross of Stone Ridge, New York; and Dr. Robert R. Shomer of Teaneck, New Jersey. Thanks also to William H. Sullivan, Jr., for a valuable interview.

I wish to express my appreciation to the American Veterinary Medical Association for sending me material and for reviewing my sections on veterinary schools and animal technicians. The Veterinary Medical Association of New York City was also helpful.

And lastly, my affectionate thanks to my daughter, Wendy Palitz, for her unflagging interest and her great help with research; to Lynn Faught and Ann O'Shea for their general support and help with infinite details; and to my editor Amy Ehrlich for her expert assistance and encouragement.

—PATRICIA CURTIS

Preface

You can read this book if you want to gain insight into the lives, the problems, and the training of veterinarians, or you can read it as I did, avidly, for the sheer enjoyment of it.

So many young people come to me and ask my advice about a possible career in veterinary medicine. I wish I could put Patricia Curtis's book into the hands of all of them.

Animal Doctors is much more than a work on careers. Such publications can be dry and boring, but Ms. Curtis feeds her information to us beguilingly, through the mouths of veterinarians of all types working in many different fields. Every branch of the profession is covered in this way, and to me, a practicing veterinarian of thirty-five years' experience, each chapter pulses with truth, with sincerity, and with the humor that is somehow bound up with the treatment of animals.

Ms. Curtis points out the pitfalls without destroying the inspiration. But make no mistake, the pitfalls do exist.

Boys and girls who are attracted to our profession by one of the most admirable traits in human nature, the love of animals, may find that this is not enough to carry them through the realities of our work: the long, unsocial hours, the discomforts, the dirt, and the hard labor.

We learn of this other side of veterinary life from the experiences of people who are themselves involved, and young readers of the book will be able to assess their own feelings when they encounter the reactions and philosophies of working veterinarians.

It must be remembered that the profession is wonderfully varied. *Animal Doctors* brings out the wonder, the satisfactions, and the fulfillments of the whole wide spectrum, from the rough, earthy life of the country practitioner to the intellectual world of the research scientist. The men and women we meet in these different worlds are all veterinarians, all helping animals in their particular ways, all reaping the rewards which come from doing a job suited to their varying temperaments.

I wholeheartedly recommend *Animal Doctors* to all those who seek an authentic picture of a possible profession and career. I recommend it, too, to the many who will find entertainment and fascination in reading about all the different and colorful ways there are of being a veterinarian.

—JAMES HERRIOT,
author of *All Creatures Great and Small*
and *All Things Bright and Beautiful*

ANIMAL DOCTORS

*I think I could turn and live with animals, they're
    so placid and self-contained,*
I stand and look at them long and long.
*They do not sweat and whine about their
    condition,*
*They do not lie awake in the dark and weep for
    their sins,*
*They do not make me sick discussing their duty
    to God.*
*Not one is dissatisfied, not one is demented with
    the mania of owning things,*
*Not one kneels to another, nor to his kind that
    lived thousands of years ago,*
*Not one is respectable or unhappy over the whole
    earth.*

WALT WHITMAN
—Song of Myself

1. "It makes us feel good to be able to cure them."

I'm going out to fetch the little calf
That's standing by the mother. It's so young
It totters when she licks it with her tongue. . . .

—ROBERT FROST

The majority of young men and women graduating from veterinary school hope to go into practice for themselves as soon as possible. Some prefer to live in a rural area and work with large animals (that is, farm animals, mostly cows and horses); others will live in cities and limit their practice to small animals (usually dogs and cats). Still others plan to have a mixed practice and treat both. Most graduates work for an established veterinarian or an animal clinic for a few years to gain experience and save up money for the huge expense of starting their own practice.

Here are a young couple, both veterinarians, who recently opened their first practice together in a farming area of New Hampshire. Jim Whitman and Karen Bell Whitman met and married while they were students at the New York State College of Veterinary Medicine at Cornell University. Karen has just gotten her degree;

Jim graduated two years ago and worked at a veterinary clinic near Ithaca while Karen finished school.

The Whitmans live in a comfortable apartment over their clinic, which has its own entrance and waiting room. A converted shed serves as a surgery for large farm animals. The place formerly belonged to an older veterinarian who has retired; the Whitmans inherited some of his clientele and are busy building their own.

While they plan to share their practice, Dr. Karen Whitman likes to do most of the work with large animals because of her love of horses, and Dr. Jim Whitman in fact prefers dogs and cats. One of his first patients in New Hampshire, however, was a big exception. He tells us about it:

Would you believe one of my first patients here was a full-grown bull moose? Well, he wasn't exactly a patient, but he did require several "house calls."

A dairy farmer who lives near us went out to bring his cows into the barn for milking one morning, and here was this moose in the pasture with the cows. The moose didn't take off when he saw the farmer, but just moved away a bit and watched. As the cows filed into the barn to be milked, the moose at first acted as though he were going to follow, then apparently decided to wait for them in the pasture.

The next morning, he was still there, and this time he was behaving like a sultan with his harem—he was definitely becoming possessive. The cows just completely accepted him, and he even tried to follow them into the barn. As the days went on, he became more and more proprietary about his cows, and finally really threatened the farmer—shook his antlers at him and wouldn't let him come into the pasture.

So the farmer called the game warden, who went over to see, and then called us.

"How do you tranquilize a moose?" he asked me.

I had never had any experience with mooses! However, I was determined to try anything. I figured out the kind and amount of anesthesia that I would use on a horse that size, and we used a dart gun to give him the injection. When he was unconscious, we tied him up with ropes and hoisted him into a truck. Then we drove him way into the hills— a good hundred miles. The game warden made me go along, in case the moose came to during the trip. He and the farmer didn't want to be alone with that creature if the anesthetic wore off!

We drove off the road and unloaded the moose in a nice clearing by some woods, miles from anywhere. Just before we untied him and left him, the game warden painted his antlers with bright psychedelic paint—red, pink, orange, blue—because by now he was interested in this peculiar moose and wanted to keep track of him. He was sure anyone seeing a moose with psychedelic antlers would report it to him.

He didn't hear anything for four days.

When he did, it was from the same farmer with the cows! The farmer went out to get his cows for milking as usual, and there stood the moose again, back with his harem. One hundred miles in four days. And he wouldn't let the farmer even *near* his cows.

This time the game warden and I didn't take him back into the hills—we delivered him to the Boston zoo, where he made quite a hit with his fancy antlers.

I never wanted to be anything but a veterinarian. My father is a veterinarian, my uncle, my grandfather—it never occurred to me that there was anything else worth becoming. When I was a kid, the high point of my life was helping my father in his clinic on Saturdays and holidays, sometimes all summer.

"Jim," he used to say to me once in a while, "you should keep your eyes open and explore other professions too. I myself think being a veterinarian is great, but you shouldn't become one just because I am. There are other good things to do in the world."

But he knew I would never want to be anything else.

Even though I was happy and excited when I finished at Cornell and started working in the clinic near Ithaca, I was really nervous with my very first cases. Not so much when an animal was in front of me on the examining table —it was over the phone that I was uncertain. I couldn't estimate which cases could wait till morning and which should be seen right away. So I would tell people who called to bring their animals right over. As a result, I seemed to be working around the clock. Karen even found me clipping a dog's toenails one Sunday afternoon! The owner had called and said the dog seemed to be limping a little, and I was afraid not to look at it immediately. Karen was still a student, but she could understand my uncertainty. Now I would know what questions to ask to determine the seriousness of a problem, but at the time we were both afraid we might overlook important symptoms.

So far, in the two and a half years I've been practicing, I haven't seen many rare, medically unusual cases, but there sure have been a lot of challenging ones. Dogs mostly—in the country they are always getting hit by cars or by mowing machines, and they are brought in all broken and mangled, with their bones sticking out. It makes you feel good when you put them back together and get them well.

I had one really weird case—a collie with a hormonal deficiency that caused his fur to fall out in huge patches and not grow back. He was healthy and well except for that, because we gave him injections of the hormones he needed every few months. But he looked so strange that people stared at him. His owners got him a warm red turtleneck sweater, which they put on him on cold winter days. The last time I saw him he was doing fine. Twenty-five years ago an animal with that medical problem would surely have died.

One thing I've learned is always to answer my clients' questions fully, no matter how difficult, or dumb, or—in some cases—funny. Some weeks ago, for example, a lady brought a six-week-old puppy in for a checkup. It was the first puppy she'd ever owned. I examined him, and he was a real healthy little pup.

But in the course of the conversation, the lady said, "You know, Doctor, he does seem to have one problem that worries me."

"Well, what's that?" I asked.

"He doesn't seem to know how to urinate," she said hesitantly. "As a male dog, he should lift his hind leg, but he only wants to pee squatting down like a female dog. I've been trying to teach him the right way. When I take him out for his walks, I tie a rope around one of his hind feet, and then I lead him up to a tree and lift his leg with the rope, so he's in the right position for a male dog to be peeing in. But he doesn't seem to catch on! Do you think he's sick?"

I'm happy to say I was able to keep a fairly straight face. I told her that *all* pups urinate that way, and that when he got bigger and more mature, he would lift his leg.

We sure do meet all kinds!

One of the advantages of our joint practice is that Karen and I can cover for each other to give us both a little free time. One day she wanted to go shopping in town, and since my case load wasn't heavy right then, I said I'd take her calls. Well, around noon one of her clients telephoned —sick cow, he said; could I come over?

The dairy farmers who are our clients here in New Hampshire range from very prosperous to not-so-prosperous, and this fellow is one of the latter. His ramshackle barn is built in two stories on a slope, with the cow stalls on the second story. You can see the lower floor right through the floorboards of the upper story.

The cow I had been called to see had milk fever (a lack of blood calcium that makes a cow very weak); she required an injection of calcium. She was in a small, awkwardly arranged stall, lying down with her head in one corner. I had to climb over the manger to reach her properly. So I'm struggling there in the stall to get the needle ready to go into her jugular vein, and all of a sudden the floor collapses. Down go the cow and I, and we're stuck, wedged together halfway through a hole in the floor, with our legs dangling in midair!

I realized I wasn't hurt, but I sure felt ridiculous, being stuck in the air with a cow. The cow apparently didn't like being there with me, either, so she started mooing, and I'm trying to get loose and climb back up to the upper story. Of course, the farmer laughed—which at the time annoyed me no end.

I had to stay that way and not try to free myself, because we were afraid the cow would fall on down to the floor below and break a leg if I got out of the hole. After the farmer brought help and tied some ropes around her, I pulled myself back up to the second story, and then we got her up.

Karen and I had a good laugh about it later. But I hope that guy fixes his rickety floor before she or I have to go back there again.

Now Karen speaks:

I was one of those typical little girls who was really crazy about horses. I joined a Four-H Club that specialized in horse activities. We went to breeding farms and horse shows and learned about horse care and equipment, how to saddle and bridle, and many other things. A lot of the girls had their own horses; I got a mare when I was in junior high, and took complete care of her myself. I think that's how I first became interested in becoming a veterinarian. Jim and I plan to get a couple of saddle horses as soon as we get established here.

When I first went to Cornell, I was a little uneasy about being in a school with mostly boys. I thought they might give the girls a hard time. But it hardly ever happened. Oh, a lot of teasing goes on—the boys ask the girls if they need any help for the few jobs that require a certain amount of physical strength, and stuff like that. But few real put-downs from the boys—and none, not any ever, from the professors. The number of girls in veterinary school at Cornell is increasing fantastically—it more than quadrupled just while I was there.

It is very exciting for Jim and me, being married and working in the same field. At first I was afraid Jim would treat me as an inferior professionally because he'd had two more years of experience. But there has never been any competition between us—we back each other up. In fact, one of the benefits of our partnership is that we are managing to avoid first-year-itis because we have each other for consultation and support. First-year-itis is the trouble most young vets get into along about the end of the first year of private practice. We come out of veterinary school wanting to lick the world and cure every disease. But those who go right into private practice alone find they have heavy case loads before they are really ready. Handling emergency cases all by yourself is especially scary. The pressure begins to build up. Then these young vets start snarling at clients.

One of my friends, whose husband is a veterinarian just completing his first year of private practice, described the symptoms of first-year-itis this way: "I knew Steve was cracking under the strain," she wrote me, "when a chair went flying out of the kitchen door one day. He had just been on the phone with a client."

Jim and I rarely have that desperate feeling of total responsibility, because whenever either of us gets a really tough case, we can share it.

Most of the farmers here in New Hampshire seem to be able to take a woman veterinarian in stride; some are even courtly and call me their "lady vet." When I'm doing a difficult procedure on an animal, they'll often try to help. "Can you really do that by yourself?" they'll ask.

One day I was handling a troublesome birth of a calf. The cow was straining, and I was struggling, trying to pull out the calf. It was hard, but I was doing okay, and the farmer was really getting in my way. "Are you sure you don't want me to do something?" he asked for the tenth time.

"Just go sit over there and look pretty," I grunted. He laughed.

That has become sort of a joke between us. On the several visits I've made to his farm, I always tell him to go sit down and look pretty.

The funniest thing is when a farmer insists on carrying my medical bag. After I've been working with a 1,200-pound animal and am covered with sweat and manure and mud, it seems so funny to have a man gallantly pick up my little bag and walk me back to the truck, as if I were delicate and helpless. But the farmers are just trying to be nice, and I'm not offended.

Another nice thing: every so often, after I've had a long or rough job at a farm, I'll go back to my truck, and there will be a jar of homemade maple syrup on the seat, or a pail of fresh-picked blackberries.

Only a few of the farmers around here are having a hard time getting used to me. The second week after we opened our practice, a farmer called and said he had a sick cow and asked if the vet could come. When he spoke to me on the phone, he must have thought I was the vet's wife. I told him the vet would be right over. Our car was in the local garage being repaired, so all we had was the pickup, which Jim needed for an errand a couple of miles beyond this farmer's place. So he dropped me off as he went past, and I went on around to the barn. The farmer couldn't believe his eyes when I introduced myself.

"I'm Dr. Whitman," I said. "You called about your cow."

He stared at me a few minutes and then decided to lead me into the barn. "A bit young, ain't you?" was all he said.

His cow had metritis, a uterine infection that cows sometimes get after calving. The farmer leaned against a stall and watched me treat the cow. He didn't say anything, just watched.

I said his other cows that had recently had calves should be examined too, and he nodded. While I was still in the barn, Jim came back to pick me up.

"You're Dr. Whitman too, are you?" said the farmer. "Well, I'll be darned."

Then, while I went to put my bag in the truck, he took Jim aside. Jim reported to me later that he said, "Your wife told me my cow had metritis."

"Then I guess that's what your cow has," said Jim pleasantly.

"She said to give her this medicine," whispered the farmer.

"If that's what Dr. Karen Whitman prescribed, you better do it," Jim told him, smiling.

The cow got well, all right, but the next time I went to this farmer, Jim happened to be along again, and the farmer still checked out what I did and said with him. Next time I'll fool him—I'll make sure to go by myself, so he'll have to take my word for whatever it is. Maybe eventually I'll win him over.

We never seriously considered practicing in a city because we both love the country so much. The only drawback I can already see is that people can't or won't spend as much money on their animals as city people do. Don't get me wrong—I'm not talking about wanting to make ourselves rich. I mean that we can't do as much for the animals as we'd like to.

All too often, the owners won't call you or bring in an animal unless it is really seriously sick. By the time you see it, it has been sick for some time, or has had an injury that has become infected because it wasn't treated. Nothing is more discouraging than trying to treat a half-dead animal! I expect we will lose many that we could have cured quite easily if we had seen them in time. I almost lost a goat with acute metritis the other day. The owner is a very good goat breeder, but even so, delayed rather long in calling me.

Another limitation is that if an animal requires expensive treatment or surgery, the owners are so quick to say, "Put it to sleep." City people seem to be more willing or more able to spend money if their pets have a good chance.

Jim's father practices in a large city, and I've seen him do amazing things to save an animal. He can do all sorts of sophisticated procedures because the owners are willing to pay for them. Here, even when you can practically guarantee that the animal will recover, it is often difficult to get the owner's agreement for you to work on it.

At veterinary school, we tried to save all sorts of creatures. I remember one spring, the first robin I saw was brought in by somebody who found it on the ground with its eyes glued shut from infection. It couldn't fly, of course. Well, our ophthalmology professor prescribed eye drops, and the robin's eyes cleared up just fine. But right then, we had a late blizzard, and while we were waiting for the weather to clear so we could release it, the poor thing died anyway. Like most wild creatures, it wouldn't eat in captivity. We all felt let down.

If you had visited our place a few weeks ago, you would have seen a beautiful horse that was practically a pet, following us around like a dog whenever he was out of the barn. I wish I could tell you he was my horse, but he was a patient we'd acquired with a lot of excitement.

One day there was a collision a few miles from our house that involved two trucks and a horse trailer. The two vehicles were damaged, and though the drivers were not seriously hurt, it looked bad for the show horse that was in the trailer. The horse was trapped in there, thrashing around and bleeding badly. The state troopers arrived and surveyed the situation. Since the wreckage blocked the highway, they wanted to get it out of the way as quickly as possible. Their solution was to shoot the horse while it was still in the wreckage and bulldoze the mess off the road.

The poor woman who had been driving the trailer when the truck smashed into it was simply beside herself. It was her horse, and she was crazy about him—he was a great horse, and a winner. But she didn't know how badly he was hurt, nor was there any way to examine him while he was in the wreckage. When I arrived, she was in tears, pleading with the troopers not to shoot the horse until the veterinarian saw it. You can imagine how I went over big with the officers, too.

"Okay, we'll give you thirty minutes to get that animal out of the trailer," the trooper in charge finally said.

I got a tranquilizer and climbed up on the wreckage, so that I could reach in and inject the poor horse. There sure was a lot of blood, but in itself that wasn't necessarily fatal. When he quieted down, all the bystanders helped me, and we literally pulled the tangled trailer off the horse in pieces. When I could get his bridle, I pulled and he struggled to his feet. He had a bad cut on his head—and as any head wound bleeds a lot, that was the cause of most of the blood.

Fortunately, at that moment Jim arrived. As soon as I'd seen there was a chance to get the horse out of the wreck, I'd asked a driver at the scene to go to our place and ask Jim to come with the trailer. We walked the horse into our van and drove him carefully to our clinic.

Do you know, all he had was that bad cut on his head, which I stitched up, and some lacerations and bruises? No internal injuries and not one broken bone. (His owner had wrapped his legs very well for traveling, and that saved his legs, I'm sure.) And those troopers were going to shoot him on the spot.

The horse spent several weeks with us, recovering. The owner visited him a couple of times, and finally he could go home with her. He'll be well enough to compete in horse shows again in a couple of months.

I'd be kidding you if I gave you the impression that every case ends as happily as those I've told you about. Sometimes you lose an animal. Often you know what it is suffering from, and you try to save it, but you were called too late, or the animal was not strong enough to begin with. The worst losses are those that you don't even know the cause of.

One day when I was covering for Jim, some people brought in a dog that seemed to be suffering from some kind of allergy. I wasn't sure. I gave it a low dose of steroid by injection to relieve the symptoms and asked the owners to bring the dog back in a few days so I could see how it reacted. Jim agreed he would have done the same thing. But next day, they brought the dog in, in convulsions— and while I was trying to save it, it died. I know the owners thought I had killed him with the steroid injection. That could not possibly have caused the dog's death, but although the people were nice about it, I know they didn't believe me. They wouldn't allow me to perform an autopsy —examine its body—to find out what had actually caused the animal's death. I lay awake all night afterward, thinking about it.

The people we deal with as veterinarians are usually under some degree of emotional strain. They have an involvement with their animal, or they wouldn't be seeing us in the first place. They may be farmers with a herd of milk cows they know intimately, or hog farmers with only a financial involvement with their hogs, or pet owners who think of themselves practically as parents of their pets. You have to remember their feelings at all times, even when you are having a hard day, and they are exasperating you with what seem like unreasonable demands.

In the long run, though, I find that most people who come to us with their animals are nice. And the satisfaction I get when I'm able to help the animals—well, I think I have the best job in the world for an animal lover!

2. "When you're out there in the jeep in some farmer's pasture, you're it."

I will not change my horse with any that treads. . . .
When I bestride him, I soar, I am a hawk.
He trots the air; the earth sings when he touches it.

—WILLIAM SHAKESPEARE

The job of a country practitioner taking care of farm animals is often rough, usually dirty, and sometimes dangerous—but it's also full of great satisfaction. The veterinarian who loves country life can have independence and challenging work, much of it outdoors.

Jack Montalvo specializes in large-animal veterinary medicine in an Eastern dairy community. He maintains an office in the big comfortable house where he lives with his wife and two small children. But the clinic where he treats his cow and horse patients is a barn or pasture; his equipment is the few tools in the bag he carries with him when he drives his jeep to the farmers and breeders who call him.

When I set up practice here eight years ago, one local veterinarian had just moved out west, and another was semiretired, so it looked as though I had a good chance to make a go of it fairly quickly. That has proved true—I even have a partner now. But I never would have guessed it from my first case. My phone rang on a chilly, misty Friday night.

"I've got a heifer down," said a dairy farmer named Anderson, who lived nearby. "Can you come over?"

When a farm animal lies down and doesn't—or can't—get up, it usually means trouble. So the words "cow down" or "horse down" will bring the veterinarian on the run.

When I got to his place, Anderson turned me over to his "manager," a kid about eighteen years old, who led me some distance out to the barn with a flashlight. The heifer was down, all right, and nearly out. She was breathing irregularly and with difficulty—what they call Cheyne-Stokes breathing. I didn't know what she had, but I knew where she was going. It wasn't the kind of case that you could call a practice-builder.

"This heifer is dying," I said to the manager. "I'll give her some fluids, but I think it's too late." And as I was putting the tube into her vein, she died.

"What do you mean, she died?" said the farmer when I told him. "She was okay this morning—she was even eating! What the devil did you do to her?"

I tried to tell him that she was nearly gone when I got to her, and asked permission to perform an autopsy to discover what she had actually died of. In an autopsy, you cut the body open to investigate the cause of death. But Anderson was so upset, he just ushered me out to my car then and there.

Well, that was bad enough, but there was more to come. Several weeks later, I was in the hardware store in our village when another farmer I knew slightly came up to me and boomed out, "Say, I hear you killed a cow up at Anderson's!"

"Who told you that?" I asked him, really taken aback.

"The artificial breeder," he said.

I happened to know that the artificial breeder was the purveyor of gossip for the whole area. He went to every farm and knew everybody's business and spread the news around. So thanks to him, I had this great reputation already.

Naturally, Anderson didn't call me again for about a year, but then one day he had an emergency and couldn't get anybody else. I got a call to get out there quick. As I drove up, Anderson came running across the pasture yelling at me to hurry. I grabbed my bag and ran after him. Clear at the end of the pasture, there was one of his cows down—down in the stream, in fact.

Now when a cow goes down, she finds the lowest land, the thickest brush, the deepest stream, head down, tail up —I mean, it's just her nature. This particular cow had milk fever, I could see right away. Milk fever is bad, but if a cow's still alive when you get there, you can treat her, and recovery can be sudden and dramatic. She was alive, and I thought to myself, "Here's my chance to win Anderson back."

So I gave her the injection for milk fever, with Anderson looking on suspiciously. By God, in a matter of minutes, that cow got up and beat us back to the barn!

When I first got out of veterinary school, I was very brave and gung ho—nothing was too dangerous for me. There is a lot of excitement in treating cows and horses— it has to do with the massiveness of the animals. But I've learned that the best way to handle them is to outwit them.

I'm too valuable to myself to play the cowboy. For example, I made up two safety rules for myself. One is, never go into a horse stall alone. I make sure to have the owner with me, and if possible I have him bring his animal out into the barn. You never know when a horse might panic and begin to rear and kick; if you're alone in the stall with it, you can get hurt.

My other rule is, never vaccinate a calf for Bang's disease when I'm alone. I must have help. It sounds funny, but vaccinating calves is one of the most dangerous things I do—not because calves can hurt you, but because the serum for Bang's disease is extremely potent. You have to give it subcutaneously (under the skin) rather than into the muscle, which means the needle is close to the surface and close to your hand. If the calf jumps, one slip of that needle, one prick of that needle into your own hand, and you're a very, very sick man.

You don't need brute strength to be a country veterinarian, but you do need endurance. Someone asked me if I thought a girl could be a large-animal practitioner, and I said I couldn't see why not, if she was healthy and had stamina. The thirty or forty pounds' difference in weight between a man and a woman isn't going to amount to much when you're dealing with a 1,500-pound animal.

A lot of youngsters around here like to ride with me on my calls, and I enjoy having them. I would advise any student who is thinking of becoming a veterinarian to spend three days, twenty-four hours a day, with a large-animal practitioner to see what it's like. In that time, a kid could probably see both the thrills and the drudgery.

Every so often, my work includes all the excitement of solving a mystery. Early one morning, I was just leaving to help a cow in a difficult labor when I got a call from a farmer named Bill Short. He was all upset—he'd been out to look at his heifers and found one dead and two staggering. Could I come right away? So, I got my partner to go deliver the cow in labor, and I jumped in my jeep and hurried out to Short's.

I took a look at the two dead heifers—a second had died while I was on the way—and all I could think of was some type of acute poisoning. I started giving the sick one methylene blue, which helps in poison cases, but she died while I was treating her.

"Get in the jeep and let's take a ride around your pasture," I said to Short.

We drove out, and the place began to look like a battlefield—a dead heifer over there under a tree, another near the fence, one still twitching by a clump of bushes. Short had had fifteen heifers in the pasture, his entire replacement herd for the year, and they were dying like flies.

Here's where a terrific feeling of responsibility comes in, a feeling all country veterinarians share, I think. When you're in small-animal practice, you have all your diagnostic aids—you can take an X ray, use your microscope, call a consultation. You can say to the animal owner, "Excuse me a minute," and go back to your books for an answer. But when you're out there in the jeep, you're *it*. You're really on the line.

So I'm driving along thinking, "All right, Montalvo, you'd better *do* something." I was in as deep trouble as I'd ever been, and I had better think quickly.

Down in the corner of the lot was the farmer's dump. "Come on," I said to Short, and we piled out of the jeep and began to search it for batteries or anything else that could cause poisoning. We found paint cans, but latex paints—harmless. The only thing to do, I decided, was autopsies—immediately. So Short and I laid the dead heifers in a row, and I got out my knife.

Well, sure enough, there in the stomach of the first heifer—a stick of dynamite! I went right down the line of heifers, and that was it, all right—acute nitrate poisoning. Back to the dump we went, and this time we found it— a paper bag, all trampled open, with a few half-chewed-up sticks of dynamite still left. It's not the most glamorous way to practice veterinary medicine, searching a farmer's dump, but boy, I was as relieved as I've ever been. I quickly gave injections of methylene blue as an antidote to those heifers that were poisoned but still alive.

"How did you happen to have dynamite in your dump?" I asked Short on the way back.

Short thought a minute. "You know, I was cleaning out the barn last week, and I came across that bag of dynamite. I'd had it for years and years. I thought I ought to get rid of it before it caused any trouble."

I put my hand on Bill Short's shoulder. "I guess you didn't find the right place to throw it away."

When a cow gives birth, the farmer usually assists himself, and only calls you in when there's trouble. Unfortunately, even then he'll often delay, and by the time you get there, the poor cow has lost all the birth fluids and has been straining so long that the calf is dead inside her, and she is nearly dead herself.

When a calf is born normally, it dives out, head and forelegs first. But when the calf presents its rump or back or a hind leg first, you have to reach in there and turn it around yourself. Or the cow may be having twins and trying to push both out at once. Sometimes, you even have to saw up a dead calf inside the mother to get it out. You can overcome most birth complications if you can train your farmer clients to call you in time, rather than waiting until the situation gets really critical.

The most disheartening call a country veterinarian can get in the middle of the night is for a cow with a prolapsed uterus. Sometimes, after too many deliveries, an older cow's uterus is weakened, and it begins to hang out like a pink bag. If you're lucky, you get there when it has just happened, and then you give the cow a spinal anesthetic and stuff the uterus back in carefully, like putting pickles in a jar.

But more than likely, things are a mess when you arrive —the cow is lying down, straining, and the uterus is filthy with manure and other dirt. You have to lie down and go to work, and you're in for a long haul. You get exhausted, itchy with dung, your arms scratched up—and you begin to think it's hopeless, you're never going to get the uterus back inside that cow. After several hours, you start thinking of all the things you can say to the farmer: How good a cow is she? Does she milk well all the time? Does she breed well? You think, maybe you can give up and persuade the farmer to slaughter her, bleed her out for meat, and you can go home.

But then you stand up, go and wash, take a break, and begin again. You can't just walk out. And eventually you get the uterus back in, and the cow nearly always becomes healthy again.

In my experience, there are two kinds of commercial farmers: the one who wants you to take care of his cows but doesn't want to spend any money, and the farmer who would hock everything he has, including his wife, to take care of his cows. The second kind usually knows his cows better than he knows his wife, no kidding. When one of his herd is sick, he knows right away.

"She's just not right," he'll say. He notices if she feels cool, if she's not letting her milk down right, if she comes in the barn out of order. Cows always come into the barn in the same order, you know—the boss cow first, then the others, according to the pecking order of the herd.

One thing the large-animal veterinarian has to compete with these days is the fact that the farmer or manager can give so much treatment himself. He can get penicillin, live vaccines—and he usually misuses them. I know one farmer who gives every cow in his herd penicillin the minute it looks cross-eyed. As a result, this farmer's cows get the worst metritis and mastitis—infections of the uterus and the udder—in the county. Horse owners make the same mistake. When an animal is overtreated with antibiotics, it builds up a resistance to them; then when it does get an infection, the antibiotic won't take effect.

Sometimes the veterinarian is called to verify a diagnosis the owner has already made and treated—and botched up. I try to persuade my clients it's better to call me unnecessarily than too late. If they tell me what's going on, I can often anticipate trouble and save their animal. Or, occasionally, it's the other way around—I can judge when it's okay to wait or do nothing. The other day one of my clients, a gentleman farmer, called me in great alarm because one of his horses was cast—that means the horse had lain down in his stall and gotten stuck with his legs folded under him. He was in such a position next to the wall of his stall that he had no room to roll onto his chest and push his weight onto his legs to get up. A cast horse can exhaust itself, and even hurt itself, but nearly always it'll get itself up eventually.

In this case, the man had gone out to the barn to feed the cats and had heard this tremendous thumping and thrashing about. When he investigated, he discovered his horse's predicament. I told him to go back to the barn and take another look, and then call me back. If the horse wasn't up, I'd come over. Ten minutes later he called, and it was as I had expected—the horse was on his feet again and okay.

One time I had an exciting piece of surgery on a valuable show horse—in fact, it was a little bit too exciting. The owners thought it was dramatic because we operated right on the lawn with all of them there, but they don't know to this day how dramatic it really was.

My patient was a six-year-old palomino named Teddy, a real big horse, and gentle. The Hardings' thirteen-year-old daughter, Lynn, was crazy about him, rode him all the time, and showed him in local horse shows. Teddy developed a lump on his neck, under the skin but attached next to the larynx, right where the jugular vein bifurcates, or divides. I had tried some treatments and procedures on the lump, but nothing had helped reduce it. I didn't want to do surgery because of its location, but I finally decided it had to come out.

I was rather nervous about the operation. It's bad enough when you lose a farmer's cow, but in this small, horsey community, a lot of horse lovers would hear about it if I botched up this particular surgery. Around here, show horses bring their owners both pleasure and money, and Teddy was the darling of this family, for sure.

I chose the broad grassy lawn between the owner's pasture and the driveway to the house as our operating room —it was cleaner there than in the barn, with more room and better light. And I picked a cool, sunny day with no wind. It was autumn, and the maple trees were vivid red and yellow. My partner, Dave Silver, and I got everything ready.

"Okay, you can bring the patient out now," I said to Lynn. One thing about being a country veterinarian—you usually have the animals' owners looking over your shoulder while you work. They're there all the time, to see your expressions, hear your comments. You can't operate in privacy before office hours, as small-animal vets do.

Dave and I had decided to use glyceryl guiacolate—a muscle relaxant—to put the horse down. Dave gave him a shot in the shoulder muscle. We motioned the family out of the way, but Dave and I stood close enough to try to guide the direction of Teddy's fall when he went down. Naturally, we wanted him to fall on his left side, because the lump was on the right side of his neck. He collapsed very nicely, and lay there full length on the grass, but as luck would have it, on his *right* side. It took Dave and me and Mr. Harding and his son Matthew to tie ropes to Teddy's feet and pull his 1,200 pounds of deadweight over to the other side. Then Dave began to give the anesthesia in the vein of Teddy's neck. We picked a slow-acting one that gives a smooth recovery. A large animal coming out of anesthesia can be extremely dangerous: it thrashes around and can hurt itself—and you. In fact, you can get yourself killed.

I spread clean towels around the area where the incision would be, knelt down, put on sterile gloves, and went to work. The Hardings, even Lynn, stood by quietly; nobody went in the house.

The lump appeared to be a tumor and was enlarged to the size of a small grapefruit, encased in a membrane, and attached. I was working as quickly as I could, trying to get it loose, when all of a sudden there was an unusually large gush of blood from the incision.

"Oh my God, I think I've cut the jugular vein!" I said to myself. "Well, Montalvo, you've had it. This horse is just plain going to bleed to death here and now." And I muttered to Dave, "We're in trouble."

Both of us tried to look cool as we worked to stop the

bleeding. But then I realized I had only cut the artery that fed the tumor.

"Whew!" Dave and I glanced at each other with relief. I clamped the artery and sewed it up, and soon I was able to lift the tumor out of the horse's neck. I put it on a tray on the grass, and then—breathing more easily—sewed up the eight-inch wound.

"Now comes an important part of the operation," I said. "Lynn, would you please come over here and sit on Teddy's head?"

"What?" gasped Lynn.

"That's right," I told her, and I motioned Mr. Harding to come over too. "Both of you lean on the head with all your weight. Teddy will be coming out of the anesthetic soon, and the first thing he'll do is try to lift his head. If he gets his head up, he'll try to stand. It is absolutely essential that he *not* stand up until he's fully awake, because he could keel over and break a leg."

I flipped Teddy's lip back and forth with my finger. The lip was lax.

"I'm testing muscle tone," I explained. "When a horse is completely under, all his muscles are relaxed, but as he comes to, he'll regain muscle tension."

After a while, Teddy's lip indicated that the anesthetic was wearing off, and he opened his eyes. Sure enough, he immediately tried to lift his head and get to his feet, but Mr. Harding and Lynn pressed him firmly to the ground. His eyes closed again, and he drifted off for a few more minutes.

Finally I said, "Okay, you can get up off him now, but get out of the way fast." We all sprang back, and just in time.

Teddy struggled to his feet. I held his bridle, and Dave grabbed hold of his tail, and between us we held the horse upright and steadied him as he staggered around. He was very groggy. When he stopped wobbling, we led him slowly around for about an hour. When he could stand firm on his legs, we let Lynn lead him back to the barn.

Dave told me afterward that cars going by on the road during the operation all slowed down while the occupants gaped out the windows. We must have been an interesting sight there on the lawn.

I sent the tumor off to the lab for tests; it was not malignant.

Teddy made a good recovery, and a few weeks later Lynn started riding him again. He's doing fine; he and Lynn took a ribbon in a horse show recently.

3. "I had childhood fantasies about taking in stray animals."

If you pick up a starving dog and make him prosperous, he will not bite you. This is the principal difference between a dog and a man.

—MARK TWAIN

A veterinarian's practice can be and usually is busy and exciting. It can also be financially rewarding. However, the profession offers a wide range of choices.

Here is a woman who loves her work but wants to lead a quiet life with little tension. She has arranged what for her is a perfect balance of professional and private life.

Elizabeth Nordstrom became a veterinarian thirty years ago, the only woman in a class of forty students at New York State College of Veterinary Medicine at Cornell University. She lives today in the green Wisconsin countryside with her youngest daughter, a college student. Dr. Nordstrom's modest clinic is just off the kitchen of her simple, cozy house. She limits her practice to dogs and cats, has a reputation for good surgery. "I'm known for my two-stitch spays," she laughs—meaning that she can spay a cat through an incision so small that it will need only two stitches.

She feels she has a completely satisfying life. It didn't happen all at once.

One June evening, I was just sitting down to read the paper after dinner at the end of a rather depressing day. I had had several cases of badly neglected animals, one poor cat with a serious urinary infection, and lastly a dear old female dog with breast cancer that had to be put to sleep. I rarely put animals to sleep—I hate it—but in this case it was unquestionably the only thing to do. So I was musing over the newspaper and enjoying the quiet when the bell to my clinic door rang.

There stood a boy about twelve years old whom I recognized as one of a family that lives about half a mile from me. Billy, this youngster's name was.

"Can you do something for this baby raccoon?" he asked me. "I found it in the woods all by itself, no mother anywhere near. It's in a bad way." He held it up for me to see.

That baby raccoon was one pitiful sight. Its face was full of porcupine quills! One quill had almost pierced an eye; the others were embedded in one cheek and all around its little nose. It couldn't have been more than three or four weeks old.

"Come in and let me see what I can do," I said, taking the small creature from Billy. I put it on my table under a strong light, and Billy held it while I took out the quills as gently as possible. "I suspect his mother abandoned him because she couldn't nurse him with all these porcupine quills in his face. I hope this one eye isn't permanently damaged. He must have gotten hit the first time she led him out of the den." After I got all the quills out, I put some antiseptic on the wounds.

I go out of my way to discourage children from picking up any wild animals in the woods. Even though we haven't had a reported case in our area for many years, there is always the danger of rabies. This creature was so very young that the chances of his being out of the den long enough to have had contact with any other animal seemed slight. Nevertheless, I cautioned Billy to be very, very careful in handling the tiny raccoon, and told him to call me if he showed any signs of illness.

"Do you think he'll live, Doc?" asked Billy.

"If you take good care of him, he has a chance," I answered. "You'll have to feed him milk around the clock until he gets old enough to eat by himself. Let's see if he'll eat something now."

I warmed some milk, got a clean medicine dropper, and showed the boy how to feed the baby raccoon, who drank eagerly. "If your sister has a doll bottle, it would be even better," I said. "Just warm the milk slightly—not too hot." Billy seemed to get a kick out of feeding the little animal.

"Phone me in a few days and let me know how he's doing," I told him, as he left with his new pet snuggled in the pocket of his jacket.

The baby raccoon not only lived but thrived. He became a real pet and followed Billy around like a dog. When he got old enough, I gave him all his shots. Once when I stopped at Billy's house, the raccoon and the family cat were playing together, rolling and chasing each other. Billy's father had to put locks on the cupboard doors near the floor because Sam, as they called him, learned to open them and get into the food.

The following spring, Billy set his pet free in the woods where he had found him, about a mile from his house. But every so often, Sam would show up at the door for a visit.

Gradually, he checked in less frequently. Last time I saw Billy, he said Sam hadn't turned up for about a year; I guess he's leading his own life somewhere in those woods.

When I was a little girl, I used to have fantasies about the animals I was going to have when I grew up. My father was dead, we lived with my grandparents in the East, and although I was crazy about animals, I wasn't allowed to have many pets. I remember once they did give me a puppy. I was ecstatic—but three days later it died of distemper. And once I had a little black cat that had been injured, and we weren't able to housetrain it. Very soon, it disappeared; I found out later my grandmother had disposed of it.

So I used to dream that when I grew up I would live in a great big house with many, many dogs and cats, and they would all have their own rooms and belongings and whatever special foods they wanted, and we would all be so happy. I planned also to have a huge barn and pasture where old, worn-out, unwanted horses would live out their days in bliss. (I guess I had read *Black Beauty* a hundred times.) In my fantasy, I could take in every homeless animal I met, and it would grow fat and sleek and happy.

Maybe my ideas about veterinarians formed vaguely then, but I do remember a specific incident that really locked me into the conviction that I was going to become one. This happened when I was about eleven.

We were visiting a farmer friend of my grandfather's. One bitter-cold early spring evening, a sow farrowed out in the barnyard, and the newborn piglets were literally freezing to death as fast as they were being born. When the farmer discovered this, we all pitched in and brought the piglets into the house, held them over the big old-fashioned stove, and rubbed them with towels and rags.

We succeeded in saving most of them. Holding those little frozen creatures and bringing them to life with my very hands gave me a strange excitement, an almost spiritual feeling. I've never forgotten it. I knew then that I had to become a veterinarian.

My mother and grandparents tried to discourage me at first. After all, this was in the 1930s—women veterinarians were still looked upon somewhat as freaks. Didn't I want to become a nurse instead? they asked me. Or a teacher?

But I was a stubborn child, and once my mother saw how determined I was, she supported me. When I was in high school, she arranged for me to visit a local veterinarian regularly and watch him work. He also encouraged me. I was accepted at the agriculture school at Cornell, and a year later was admitted to the veterinary college. There were 400 applicants that year, and they took forty.

I had heard that in some of the lab courses, the male students grumbled about having to work with a female lab partner, and there I was, the only girl in my class. I was apprehensive at first. But the boys were nice—I always had a lab partner. In fact, throughout veterinary college, it was like having thirty-nine brothers.

The veterinary college at Cornell was founded long ago by a Scotsman named Law, I think it was, and when I was there, his four daughters—by then old ladies in their eighties and nineties—were still living in Ithaca. It was their custom once every year to invite all the women veterinary students to tea. So four times during my years in veterinary school, I went to tea with several other girls at the Law sisters'. They were lively little old ladies; I was surprised that none of them had become veterinarians.

We mainly studied the horse. In those days, there was no such thing as specializing in large or small animals. In the entire four years, every student performed only two spay operations; this turned out to be a big handicap to me later.

I remember only one problem that came up because I was female. The women students were not allowed to take tours of night duty at the veterinary service run by the college or ride ambulatory clinic on emergency calls to the surrounding farms. That's because it was unthinkable for a woman student to be out of the dormitory all night! Girls were closely chaperoned at college back then, restricted by all sorts of "protective" rules. So we women vet students wound up missing a very practical part of our training.

I got married my senior year, to an engineering student. When we graduated, we moved to St. Louis, where my husband had a job. To my dismay and disappointment, I could not find work. I hunted and hunted for a position with a veterinarian, and with each rejection I lost confidence, which of course further increased my chances of being rejected. Then I began to have children, and I was faced with the option of getting someone to take care of them if I found a job, or staying home and taking full-time care of them myself. I chose to stay home, partly out of my pleasure in my children and partly out of uncertainty about myself as a doctor. Also, this was during World War II, my husband joined the Navy, and we kept moving around. Weeks would go by without my even thinking of the fact that I was a veterinarian. And it got to the point where it was a little embarrassing when people found out I was a vet and wasn't practicing.

Then the time came when one of our children needed some special, very expensive schooling. We were living in Illinois then. I tried a lot of dumb jobs because I felt so inadequate in my profession. But finally I got up my nerve and applied to the veterinarians in the area as a part-time assistant. Much to my surprise, after my disappointment earlier in St. Louis, I got a job covering the practice of a vet who had to be out of the office a good deal. He wasn't there to train me, and maybe that was good for me— being on my own. It was sink or swim. I used my books and my common sense, and gained confidence. Gradually, I began to be called more and more, until I was covering for maybe ten other veterinarians.

"I'll try anything but surgery," I always said. I had a real fear of attempting surgery. Most veterinarians take an internship or apprenticeship right after graduation and get some supervised experience, but I hadn't had that. I didn't want to take on someone's pet and mess up. So I always referred any surgical cases that came in to other vets.

Then we moved to Madison, Wisconsin, and since my children were old enough by that time to be independent after school, I began to work full time for a veterinarian who had a very busy clinic. This veterinarian also ran an animal foundling hospital; stray cats and dogs who were not claimed or adopted after five days had to be put to sleep. One day I had an idea.

"Doctor," I said to my boss, "could I try spaying some of these animals that are going to have to be destroyed anyway? I need the experience, and if one dies, at least it won't be someone's pet."

"Go ahead," he said.

So I started spaying stray female cats and dogs right and left. I picked young animals, and if any of them needed other surgical procedures, I did those, too. It was hard, really hard, getting up the nerve, but I just decided it was now or never.

Much to my relief, every animal I operated on lived. So

then I would take them home and put them up for adoption. I'd run an ad in the paper, and when people found out I was giving away pets that were already neutered, I had no trouble placing them in homes. Meanwhile I found I was pretty skillful at surgery and enjoyed it!

It's a good thing I had that experience, because my husband died, leaving me with three teenagers to support. I bought an old house in a small town—right on the main street, where I was easily accessible—and opened my own practice. I supported myself and the kids well, but nearly worked myself to death. I was even taking calls for large animals—horses and cows! I thought of opening my own hospital and even went back to school and took a course in small-animal hospital management. I hired several assistants and was on my way to having a really thriving veterinary practice.

Then I got sick, mainly from overwork. And when I was on my feet again, I decided I either had to expand my facilities and hire a lot of help, or do what I really wanted—live out here in the country and have a practice just big enough for me and one part-time assistant.

I'm glad I chose this course. I now work four or five hours a day and refer any cases I can't handle to other doctors. I have just a few cages here for animals to stay overnight; I try to keep things simple for me and as inexpensive as possible for the clients. This is an economically depressed part of the state, and people who love pets but don't have money to spend on them badly need a veterinarian. My overhead is low. I love what I'm doing.

Sometimes I give a talk to a PTA or a church or civic group in the area to persuade people of the urgent need to have their dogs and cats neutered. Even out here in the country, the pet population is out of control. You see stray, wild, and starving cats and dogs everywhere. So many people won't have their pets neutered, yet they can't keep all the offspring. The one local animal shelter is overflowing. I know I can't do much as an individual, but I have to try. The people in the community are beginning to listen to me. And I do my share of free castrations and spays for people who really cannot pay.

Sometimes I run into people who are surprised to find a woman veterinarian. When I answer the phone, they ask to speak to the doctor, assuming that I'm the receptionist. When I say, "I'm the doctor," there's a pause while they readjust the image they have of the person at the other end of the telephone. Only once has anyone ever hung up when he found out I was the veterinarian.

In fact, a lot of people seem happy to find a woman vet. They say they think a woman is more gentle with animals, more sensitive—and perhaps even more compassionate toward the owners.

In my experience as a vet, I see a great deal of neglect of animals, and usually there's nothing you can do about it. One of the worst types of offenders is little old ladies— for some reason it's little old ladies rather than men— who have huge collections of cats, and the animals breed and breed. The situation gets out of hand—the old ladies can't afford to feed them properly, they can't or won't have them neutered, but don't want to give them up. Then someone will complain to the ASPCA, who'll come and clean out all the cats. But the little old lady will have one or two hidden away, at least one unspayed female who's a special pet, and soon the whole process starts over again.

And then there are the college students. The first thing a kid will do when he or she gets away from home is acquire a cat or dog, or several. Some college students take wonderful care of their pets and are thoroughly responsible. But many who seem to love their pets while they have them will go home at the end of the school year and simply leave them behind. Every summer, college campuses all over the country are swarming with desperate, starving, abandoned dogs and cats.

I don't want to sound eccentric, but sometimes my diagnosis is done not through visual or tactile means, but through a kind of perception that I can't explain. Some medical doctors today believe the same thing—that they get insights or hunches, when they first look at certain patients, about what the disease might be or where to look for trouble. I seem to have it with animals. The practice of veterinary medicine, like the practice of human medicine, is part science and part art, of course, but this thing I'm talking about is more than that. You could call it intuition.

Just last week, I had a case that I think was an example of this. A man and woman brought in their big old hound dog named Hector.

"He seems to have something wrong with one of his hind legs," said the man. "He keeps holding it up in a funny way, and walks awkwardly."

"But when we looked at the leg, we couldn't find anything the matter with it, no mark or anything," the woman added. "Also, we think he's in pain. He doesn't seem himself."

"How long has he been this way?" I asked.

The couple looked at each other and pinned it down to a week or ten days. "We thought we'd better have you take a look at the old fellow." He patted the dog's head. Hector wagged his tail listlessly. He was holding his leg up, but I had a sudden hunch the problem was not the dog's leg.

"You know, I bet he's got something in his rectum," I

said. "Will one of you please hold him while I examine him?"

I put a glove on, put Vaseline on my finger, knelt down, and reached in. Sure enough, way inside, I could feel a big, round, hard mass. The dog winced in pain and tried to squirm away.

"I'll have to give him an anesthetic and get that mass out of his colon," I said. "That's what's hurting him. It feels like bones in there. He must be all blocked up, too. He probably holds his leg up in an attempt to ease the pain."

"For heaven's sake! Poor old Hector. He has always loved bones and has never had any trouble before. I didn't realize bones could harm him," said the woman. "Shall we wait for him?"

"No. Leave him and come back later in the day," I advised. "This will take a while. Bones can cause an intestinal blockage, and that's what Hector has. It's good you brought him in—he could have died."

So I put old Hector under anesthesia and started giving him enemas. It took several forceful enemas, plus a lot of working away with my finger, to break up and dislodge the mass. And of course there was a putrid accumulation of stool that the enemas washed out too. It wasn't what I would call my favorite way to spend an afternoon, giving enemas to an unconscious dog, but it saved Hector's life. When he came to, his relief was plain to see. He acted like a different dog.

When Hector's owners came back for him, I started to caution them against feeding him bones, but I didn't have to say much—they understood the danger.

The next day I had to remove a chicken bone from a kitten's throat. I guess it was my week for bones. Many people don't realize bones can kill a cat or dog.

Of course, most of the time I don't need intuition to

know what's wrong with an animal: the problems are plain to see. One day recently, a woman I had never seen before drove into my driveway and got out of her car carrying an injured puppy.

"I hit him with my car," she said, almost in tears. "I just didn't see him at the side of the road, and he got frightened, I guess, and ran right into the path of my car. Please do everything you can for him, Dr. Nordstrom. I feel so guilty!"

One of the puppy's paws was badly mashed. What also worried me was that he was so thin and weak—really emaciated, in advanced starvation. "He must have been abandoned along the road weeks ago," I told the woman. "He may have other things wrong with him too. He's a poor surgical risk, and I don't know what I can salvage of his paw."

But the woman wanted me to try. He was an appealing pup, about four or five months old, with a sweet face. It's hard to imagine what sort of person would throw him out of a car, yet people do it all the time to pets they don't want. I agreed to do my best for him. First thing I did was vaccinate him for distemper and hepatitis. Then I gave him intravenous anesthesia and supportive fluids, and took a look at his paw. I discovered two of the toes were broken off inside the skin. They were impossible to repair, so I had to remove them. The surgery was tricky, but I was pleased with the result. And he came through.

Next day, I discovered he was loaded with intestinal worms—roundworms, tapeworm, hookworms. I wormed him, cleaned him up, and then wondered if the woman who had brought him would really come back for him.

"What will I do with you if she doesn't?" I said to the dog, as I changed the bandage on his paw. He wagged his tail and tried to lick my face, in spite of the pain he must have been feeling in his paw. He was so relieved to be warm and fed, he thought his troubles were over, I guess.

But you know, early in the evening, the woman did come back.

"I haven't been able to get him out of my mind," she said to me. "I was going to pick him up from you, pay his bill, and then drop him off at the animal shelter and hope someone would adopt him. But I think I'll keep him. I think he was intended for me."

She continued to bring the dog back so that I could check on his paw, and the last time I saw him he was beginning to look great and seemed so content. That's one abandoned dog who was lucky. It was a happy ending, almost right out of my childhood fantasy.

4. "I hung out my shingle and simply made up my mind to do the very best medicine I could."

Animals are such agreeable friends—they ask no questions, they pass no criticisms.

—GEORGE ELIOT (Mary Ann Evans)

Some veterinarians take a roundabout route to arrive at their profession. Instead of studying a preveterinary course in college and then going straight into veterinary school, a few people start off in a different direction. Later, realizing what they really want to do, they manage to go to veterinary school and eventually wind up happy and busy in the type of practice that's right for them. Here is a veterinarian who has done that.

Kenneth Frary, a black man of about forty, has a thriving small-animal practice in a densely populated industrial area where many small townships merge. He is active in his state's veterinary association and also in recruitment for his alma mater, Tuskegee Institute School of Veterinary Medicine.

He speaks thoughtfully about his life and work.

"No, you can't keep him!" exclaimed my mother. It was about the hundredth time I had sneaked a dog or cat into the house. I had always wanted a pet. As far back as I can remember, I wanted a dog or cat. My mother definitely did not want one.

So when I was ten or eleven, I took to hanging around a veterinary clinic. The veterinarian tolerated me, let me help out—well, he let me sweep up the place or give the animals fresh water or some such. I watched everything he did. When I got older, he even gave me a job. I worked as a sort of kennelman—cleaned out cages, held animals while the vet examined or treated them, stayed overnight to keep an eye on especially sick ones, that sort of thing.

Then, when I was in my teens, I got a job as a handyman on a farm that had a lot of animals—horses, cows, pigs, sheep. You'd never believe it now, but there was still a lot of farmland hereabouts in those days. I worked on this farm off and on, summers and vacations, during my high school and college years.

After high school, I went down south to an agriculture college and majored in animal husbandry—that means breeding. Then I went into military service, and by the time I came out, the farmland here was mostly gone, and I could not get a job in animal husbandry in this entire state. So I worked in a shipyard.

But I wasn't happy; I knew I had to find some way to work with animals. I decided to apply to veterinary school at Tuskegee, which in those days was all black, and I was accepted. When I graduated, I came back home and looked for a job with an established veterinarian. I needed practical experience, but nobody would hire me. Some didn't need an assistant—their practice didn't warrant one. And some told me right out that they were afraid they would lose their clientele if they hired a black veterinarian. I appreciated their frankness, I could even understand their feelings, but I was beginning to get discouraged.

Then an older veterinarian in another part of the state offered me a job. He had a busy small-animal practice, and working for him gave me a great chance to get practical experience. I worked for him nearly two years.

At first I was very apprehensive. He was white, his clients were white, and I was worried that they wouldn't accept me. Well, all my fears were unfounded, because nobody dropped dead when they saw me there working for Dr. Bellow. We worked side by side. In the beginning, this frustrated me a bit—I'd had all those years of veterinary school, and I was itching to start putting my education into practice. I'd wonder, "What am I doing, just standing here holding this dog?"

But soon I understood completely. I was getting work experience with supervision and also being given the chance to earn the respect and confidence of white clients. Also, at veterinary college, I had gotten comparatively little training with dogs and cats—most veterinary education then was aimed at the care of large animals. I learned a lot from Bellow. I still believe strongly in apprenticeship or internship—it's the best way for a graduate veterinarian to learn to apply what he or she has learned in school.

After a couple of years, I thought I was ready to be on my own. Dr. Bellow offered to lend me the money to set up my own practice—I'll never forget him for that. But I came back home here and raised the money on my own. I found this building for my hospital, and my whole family and all my relatives pitched in and helped me set it up.

There had never been a black veterinarian in this part of the state. I had no idea how I'd make out. In fact, a lot of people—including my family—wondered too. But I hung out my shingle and waited to see what would happen. I simply made up my mind to do the very best medicine

I could and hoped people would like my service and tell others. I think I saw two patients the first day.

I took on large animals, too, for the few farms still left in the area. But I had a bad experience with a high-strung saddle horse that persuaded me to give up that kind of practice. The horse had a deep laceration above the fetlock that required sutures, or stitches. I took all the precautions I knew, had the horse thoroughly tranquilized—I thought. While I was bending over suturing his leg, that horse cut loose with a kick that knocked me across the stable, unconscious. When I came to, I thought, "My goodness, I've got a wife and two children—I'd just as soon give up this kind of dangerous work."

Well, as it turned out, I didn't need it anyway. Two years after I opened my animal hospital, I had to hire another veterinarian to help with my practice. That was six years ago. We get a wide variety of small-animal cases, my practice has just grown and grown, and now I plan on expanding our facilities.

My clientele is ninety-five percent white.

A typical day? Let's just take today, it was pretty typical. I started at 6:00 this morning with surgery. I had a couple of castrations, four or five spays; my partner unplugged a male cat—that means he relieved a blockage in the cat's urinary bladder.

I removed a bladder stone the size of a large orange from a middle-aged dog; he's going to be okay. But I had to remove an eye from another dog that had been in a car accident. She's in our intensive care unit now—a special cage where an animal's vital signs are monitored by machines, and where it receives oxygen and fluids; we're doing all we can, but I don't expect her to make it.

We try to complete our surgery by around 8:30, because

we open up and start seeing clients at 9:00. Our case load averages forty-five animals a day, not counting surgical cases. My partner and I schedule routine surgery—that's nonemergency cases, of course—three days a week and average ten operations on those days.

At 11:00 I go home for lunch and rest, and come back at 4:00. I try to leave by 7:00, but it's usually more like 9:00.

Because there's no one at the hospital during the night, animals that need close watching and round-the-clock care would be untended. I solve that problem by taking the very sick ones home with me in a special portable unit equipped with everything the animal might need, such as bottles and tubes for intravenous fluids. I check the animal several times during the night. I can see quickly if there's any change for the worse and take care of it. Also, I think it gives a sick animal the encouragement it needs. I believe this kind of attention can often make the difference between life and death in a very sick, dependent animal like a cat or dog.

Once I had taken a woman's cat home with me—it was quite sick and needed medication before morning. About 9:30 that evening the woman telephoned me—she apologized but said she was so worried about her pet that she had to find out if it was all right. I told her her cat was doing fine, but she sounded so upset that I said she could come on over and see for herself. So she drove to my home, paid a little visit to her cat, and went away reassured.

One of the most difficult aspects of being a veterinarian is learning how to get along with your clients, the owners of your patients. You have to allay their fears, understand their concern, and be patient.

I find it helps to be perfectly frank with them. I tell them what I'm doing with their pet and why I'm doing it, what tests I'm taking and what the results are. In my experience, the more a client knows, the better he or she can cooperate for the sake of the animal.

Your chief responsibility is to the animal. Between you and the animal stands the owner; both you and the animal need the owner to carry out the treatment you prescribe. Your best bet is to make the owner an ally, enlist his or her cooperation. No matter what pressure you're under, you have to learn to do this if you're going to be a successful veterinarian.

Another thing you have to learn in this business is that for a lot of people, pets are the same as children. Others—lonely people—rely on their animals for companionship. In an increasingly impersonal world, pets mean more and more to their owners, and some folks become very dependent on their dogs or cats to keep them company. When an animal is brought into my clinic, one thing I always take into consideration is what the animal means to the person who brings it in or how it fits into a family. Is it the only pet of a single person, or of a childless couple? Is it the pet of an older couple? Of a sportsman? Of an animal breeder? Is it a child's pet? A family pet? These are important details.

People are starved for some connection with natural life. Pets are especially interesting to urban people, who have no other opportunity to have regular contact with nature. Even when it is becoming harder and harder to keep animals in cities, the pet business is booming. That's good for us, of course, although it becomes an increasing responsibility to educate owners to take care of all their pets properly.

For example, a lot of folks think a neutering operation will change their pet somehow—make it fat, or change its personality. This is nonsense. If a cat or dog is fat, it is because its owner overfeeds it, that's all. Other people think they are depriving their animal of something by not letting it have sex. Believe me, an animal is unaware of missing anything—and in fact, a neutered or altered one is a lot more comfortable than an unaltered one.

An unaltered tom gets torn up in ferocious fights, and nobody wants him around because he sprays and smells. An unspayed female who's kept indoors howls and is clearly miserable, but if you let her out, she's doomed to repeated pregnancies, and you have the problem of destroying the kittens or finding homes for them—no easy task, these days when the animal population is at a record high. Last year, 13.5 million unwanted cats and dogs had to be put to death. What a waste of life—and also of human activity!

We need a vast birth-control program for pets. There's some research going on for birth-control pills for animals. The biggest problem, though, is to educate the public to the need for control.

The veterinarians in this area work together closely. I am active in our local veterinary society, have held several offices in it, and am also a member of a volunteer service that covers a wide area here. It's a twenty-four-hour-a-day, seven-day-a-week service; if any of our regular clients needs us for an emergency—or anybody just picks one of us out of the phone book—the answering service will give the person the name and phone number of whichever vet is on emergency duty. We take turns according to a schedule.

This service works well for the customer because it means he or she can get a veterinarian at any time, and it frees us from being on call day and night. We can go away for an evening, or even a weekend, without worrying that our practice isn't covered for emergencies. No member of the volunteer service ever tries to steal another member's clients.

Just last Sunday I was on call for our volunteer service and treated an emergency case for one of my associates. A man telephoned very upset and said he had to get his cat to a vet right away—the cat had gotten caught in a trap. I told him to bring it to my clinic immediately.

In a short time he arrived with his little daughter, a child about ten, holding a beautiful black cat in her arms. The girl was crying.

"Am I glad you're here today!" the father exclaimed. "My idiot neighbor set a trap for a rabbit he says eats the vegetables in his garden. Can you imagine setting a trap in a populated area with kids and pets running around? I found our cat caught in that thing, mewing away and bleeding. I'm afraid her paw is badly hurt." He was really angry, and I don't blame him.

The cat needed treatment immediately. She had lost quite a lot of blood and was in pain and shock. First I gave her an injection to sedate her and ease the pain. Then I administered an injection of antibiotic for infection and cleaned the wound thoroughly with soap and water. I began an intravenous drip to combat shock and X-rayed the paw to check for broken bones. Fortunately, there were no fractures, so I bandaged the paw in an antibiotic dressing, which would have to be changed daily. I wrote out a complete report for my colleague. I put down the nature of the injury, what treatment and medication I gave— everything the other vet would need to know to take it from there. And finally, I reassured the girl and gave the man some advice on how to make that darn fool neighbor get rid of his illegal trap.

If the man had had to drive some distance or wait till the next day to get medical care for that cat, his child might have lost her pet. I always find it especially gratifying to save a child's pet. Of course, my first responsibility is to the animal, regardless of who or what kind of person the owner is. If an owner is insensitive or unpleasant when I've knocked myself out for an animal, well, I just take it in stride. But children are always so appreciative, I get a big kick out of them.

5.

"At our hospital, we try to be aware of every animal's feelings."

A cat does not place its affections thoughtlessly. It wishes only to be your friend (if you are worthy of it) and not your slave. It retains its own free will and will do nothing for you that it considers unreasonable.

—THEOPHILE GAUTIER

Though the number of women veterinarians is presently small in proportion to men, their percentage is rising fast. It is predicted that in ten years some forty percent of all veterinarians will be women.

California-born Peggy MacAdam, who graduated from veterinary school six years ago, works with three other veterinarians in a busy small-animal hospital in Los Angeles. She and her colleagues have worked hard to earn the hospital a reputation for efficient teamwork and excellent animal medical care.

Dr. MacAdam lives not far from the hospital with her architect husband and their five-year-old daughter. Typical of many young professionals, they share the housework and child care.

I wanted to be an animal doctor as far back as I can remember—even before I had ever heard the word "veterinarian." I may have even believed that becoming a doctor for animals was an original idea of mine, something brand-new that nobody else had ever thought of. Then along about third grade I heard that animal doctors had already been invented and were called "veterinarians"; I was even more convinced this was my thing to do.

When I was in high school, I briefly entertained the idea of becoming an M.D. instead. I remember my grandmother encouraged me especially; I think she thought being a medical doctor had more class. But my mother always said, "You can do whatever you want." Neither she nor my father ever said, "Little girls don't become veterinarians," or any of that nonsense.

It's funny, though, how people in general still often think in terms of stereotypes. Children are conditioned early. I have two little nephews who visit me here at the clinic now and then, and they have seen me work. My daughter, of course, doesn't think what I do is at all unusual, but one day when I was visiting my sister, my nephew Nicky, the five-year-old, said to me: "Let's play doctor. I'll be the doctor and you be the nurse."

"But I want to be the doctor," I said.

"You can't be the doctor—you're a *girl*. Girls can't be doctors, they have to be nurses," my nephew explained patiently.

"But Nicky, you know I really *am* a doctor," I persisted.

Nicky thought that one over. Then he conceded good-naturedly: "Okay. We'll both be doctors."

Occasionally, in our practice here at the hospital, a new client reacts with: "*You're* one of the vets?" It may be partly because I look so young. No one has ever actually said, "I don't want you to work on my animal." I just once in a while sense a little distrust at first, almost always from middle-aged people. Young people don't see anything unusual. And old people always seem to get a kick out of the fact that I'm one of the veterinarians here.

A few people insist on having me *because* I'm a woman. I would really prefer that they ask for me because they like me.

When I was at the University of California at Davis, the preveterinary course was only two years, and I was lucky enough to get into the veterinary college after that. Some people in my class, however, had their bachelor's and even master's degree. I was one of eight women in our class of about eighty; there are many more than that now.

We need another veterinary college in California, but the public won't support a bond issue for it—mainly, I think, because they don't realize all the different things veterinarians do that affect the public: medical research, consumer protection, public health, and other vitally necessary work. The public just thinks, "My goodness, we don't need any more doctors to take care of pets!" So there is a bad shortage of veterinarians. I heard that they had 900 applications at Davis last year, and they can only take eighty students.

Some animal husbandry courses were required when I was in veterinary school, and of course I did some work with large animals. I felt quite comfortable with them then. I even once castrated a bull! Our class went out to the feedlot with our professor, and here was this bull in a chute, throwing a fit. He was snorting and bellowing and pawing the ground and really carrying on. Of course, he was squeezed in tight, so he couldn't hurt himself and theoretically couldn't hurt anyone working on him. But he was really mad.

"All right, who wants to castrate this bull?" our teacher asked.

"I do!" I said.

I was the only woman in this particular class, and it just happened that all the men were small-animal oriented. None of them said a word. The professor flipped, he thought it was so funny. Actually, because my arms are skinny, I had an advantage—I was less of a target for the bull's kicking.

I haven't worked with large animals at all since I graduated, and to tell the truth, I'm a little nervous around them now. Horses especially—one bad kick can get you a fractured skull or a ruptured spleen. But some women I know do large-animal work and love it.

When I graduated from veterinary school, it took me a while to find a job—but not at all because I'm a woman. I was just picky. For one thing, I wanted to stay in or near L.A. I wanted to work five days a week and not be exploited because I am young. But the main thing I wanted was to find a place where I could do a wide variety of jobs and really good medicine. Some veterinarians limit their practices and refer cases they don't want or aren't equipped to handle. That's okay for them, but I wanted to do just about everything. Also I didn't want to work in a place where making money was the overriding concern. This hospital is just fine for me.

My colleagues Dr. Schramm and Dr. Elliot do most of the major surgery because they really like it. I do a little soft-tissue surgery, but Dr. Devereaux and I prefer the purely medical cases—that is, the ones that don't involve surgery—so we generally handle most of those. The work here is divided and shared to everybody's liking.

Dr. Schramm served a residency at the Animal Medical Center, the famous teaching hospital in New York. During part of that time, he worked in a human hospital doing a comparative study of heart disease. Many heart diseases are very similar in animals and human beings. We give some of the same treatments, and Dr. Schramm even performs some of the same operations that save the lives of human heart patients. In fact, one of the first patients I saw when I started work here was a dog with heart disease. The owner brought in a middle-size brown dog of uncertain ancestry named Spot. At first glance, Spot didn't appear particularly sick.

"What seems to be the matter with him?" I asked.

"Nothing really bad—just a bunch of little things," said Spot's owner, a man about fifty years old wearing work clothes. "He gets tired easily, doesn't run as much when I take him for walks—he'll start to chase a squirrel and then give up, breathing hard. He's eight years old, but he was lively till recently."

"Have you noticed a cough?"

"Yes, now and then," answered the man. "But mostly it's that he's gotten lazy, sleeps a lot. Just doesn't seem to be himself. I think you better take his temperature. Maybe he's sick."

Taking Spot's temperature was not the important thing, I had already begun to suspect. However, I always do whatever a client asks, if it won't hurt the animal. Spot's temperature was normal. But when I put my stethoscope to his chest, I picked up trouble. I called Dr. Schramm in for consultation, and he confirmed my diagnosis. I asked him to prescribe because he knows more about heart disease than the rest of us.

Spot was lucky—he had an observant owner. Some people would not have noticed the symptoms of heart disease in their pet as quickly. We treated this dog with medicine, placed him on a low-salt diet to control water retention, and restricted his exercise a little so he wouldn't stress the heart. Spot got much better; we saw him from time to time, and he lived happily for almost four more years.

Cats are also subject to heart disease—at least a dozen different types. Just recently, for example, a couple brought in their beautiful Siamese cat with no symptoms except inactivity.

"He used to play wildly and run around the house chasing imaginary enemies and having a great time," said the woman. "Now he just sleeps a lot."

"His favorite toy is the cork out of a wine bottle," the man told me. "Usually if I throw it for him, he'll streak after it and bring it back in his mouth and drop it at my feet. He loves that game. But last night when I tried to play with him, he just lay on the rug and watched me throw the cork. He's got to be sick!"

Dr. Schramm let them listen to their cat's heart with his stethoscope. Even with no medical experience, they could tell that the rhythm of the heart was abnormal. We also took an electrocardiogram and an X ray of the cat's heart. It is hard to get an accurate electrocardiogram on a cat, but the X ray indicated that he had a disease of the heart muscle. Most cats live only six months to a year with this disease, but on the medication we prescribed, this cat lived for almost five years. He could even chase his wine cork again.

We are very concerned about the pet overpopulation here in Los Angeles, which is as bad as everyplace else. The animal shelters are overflowing. Many veterinarians don't think free spay clinics are the answer, and obviously the public has to be educated to think of neutering as both natural and necessary for every pet they have. But here at the hospital, we do try to help by doing free neutering of cats one night a week for low-income owners. The four of us veterinarians take turns; each of us gives up an evening once a month to spay or alter people's cats on a first-come, first-served basis. It's only a drop in the bucket, considering the enormity of the problem, but we feel we're doing something to help.

Our hospital was designed by an architecture student as her senior project, and we think it's great. It's a pleasing, comfortable, functional environment, with good details like varied lighting levels to prevent eyestrain. We even have windows where observers can watch surgery—some pet owners like to do that, surprisingly. The animals' cages are roomy, and the sicker patients are kept where we can see them all the time, all day. The whole place gets a lot of sun and is full of plants. The ventilating system is first-rate.

Any time an animal has to spend more than five to seven days in a hospital, it will begin to suffer from depression. It gets homesick. Some breeds of dogs especially —collies, afghans, salukis—lose their will to live. The problem of depression is not taught in the curriculum of any veterinary school I know of, yet I think it is a big factor in an animal's recovery chances.

We always encourage the owner to visit the pet and bring it something from home, like a favorite toy or a possession of the owner's, to keep with it at the hospital.

We make it a point to try to be aware of every animal's feelings. Some animals—cats especially—also become depressed about being dirty. When they get blood or food or feces on their fur and can't clean themselves properly, it can really bother them. They need to be cleaned regularly. Also, we go out of our way to pat our patients on the head, talk to them, fondle them, take them out for walks if they're able. The only contact some vets bother to have with their patients is to give them pills and injections and treatments; how do they expect the animals to feel about them if that's all they get from them?

One time we had an Irish setter here at the hospital for twenty-four days. One of our assistants, Amy, took this dog on as her special patient and spent time with him. She brushed him, took him for walks, brought him little treats. When that dog went home, he was bright and lively. In spite of the medical care he was getting, I am sure he would have gone steadily downhill if it hadn't been for Amy.

We cater to individual animals' tastes as much as we can. For instance, we had a very sick cat last month that wasn't eating. She needed nourishment, and we fed her intravenously for a while, and then we decided to tempt her with different kinds of food. The owner said this cat was crazy about tuna. Well, we don't feed tuna to our cats here—and we advise owners not to—because cats can get steatitis, a very serious disease, from oily fish such as tuna and salmon. But in this case, we decided to throw the rule overboard and go along with the animal a little. We offered her white meat tuna (less oily). She perked up and ate that. Gradually we mixed other food in with the tuna, and finally phased it out completely when she continued to eat. In a place like ours, which isn't too big and impersonal, we can give that kind of individual care.

Occasionally something other than a dog or cat comes into our hospital. I had a goat with lead poisoning the other day—he'd eaten some stuff with lead paint on it. Last week I had a rabbit with hairballs. I've had guinea pigs, rats, turtles, snakes.

The only thing I won't do is put a healthy animal to sleep. I don't believe in it; it goes against everything I've been taught. What I especially don't like are owners who are unwilling to spend money to cure a sick or injured pet who has a good recovery chance. People like that usually hint around, hoping I will suggest putting the animal to sleep myself. They say things like "He won't ever be really healthy again, will he, Doctor?" or "Isn't it better to put her out of her pain rather than let her suffer?" They want to be able to say it was the vet, not they themselves, who decided their animal had to be put to sleep—it would get them off the hook with their consciences.

I have a hard enough time putting an animal to sleep even when I believe it has no chance. Sometimes an animal makes it against all odds. Recently I was treating a litter of puppies that had a serious disease. The owner brought them in in a box every day for treatment, along with the mother dog. All the pups were responding except the runt of the litter, who wasn't doing well at all.

Poor tiny sick thing. I had given up hope of saving it. One day I was medicating it, and it looked so miserable and so far gone, I myself began to think it might be a kindness just to give it an overdose of anesthetic. Just then it gave a little squeal. "I'm alive!" it seemed to say. I simply couldn't do it.

When that puppy pulled through along with the rest, I was really thrilled.

My job is to defend the animal. I think all living things have a place on this earth. People are important, but not to the exclusion of other living things.

6.

"The majority of animals we share our planet with are getting a raw deal."

Those who wish to pet and baby wild animals "love" them. But those who respect their natures and wish to let them live normal lives love them more.

—EDWIN WAY TEALE,
"April 28," *Circle of the Seasons*

The veterinarian who is a horse lover has several opportunities for specialization. Thoroughbred breeding farms and racetracks employ veterinarians, and any area with a large number of privately owned horses can usually support a specialist.

Not far from San Francisco there's a rolling, grassy countryside dotted with affluent farms and ranches whose stables, corrals, and practice rings indicate "horse country." Stephen Coles is an equine veterinarian here. Dr. Coles lives in a comfortable house on four pleasant acres with his wife and three teen-age sons, three dogs, four cats, and four horses, including a beloved half-Arabian mare aged twenty-two (a remarkable age for a horse to reach). He is the author of a textbook on horse care.

Dr. Coles is an activist, using his skills and his knowledge as a veterinarian to fight abuses of animals and to try to bring about changes to protect them. He has investigated the mistreatment of horses and testified against it; he finds the time to be a participating member of several animal-protection organizations, including one for wildlife, which he founded. His humane activities take him all over the country.

Here he begins his story by telling us of his work on behalf of the mustangs of Nevada.

We drove out in a Land Rover on a dusty road across the vast, flat range that lies along the San Antonio Mountains of southwest Nevada. It is a desert area of thousands of treeless acres, with a low cover growth of poor forage plants that can survive in arid conditions. On this rugged terrain, owned by the U. S. Government, small herds of wild horses have roamed free for centuries.

Suddenly, off in the distance, there they were—a group of horses grazing in the hot sun. We were looking at some of the remaining descendants of the original Spanish horses brought to this continent by the conquistadors over four hundred years ago. Mustangs, as they are called, are a living symbol of the Old West. They belong to no one, yet in a way they belong to all Americans.

We turned off the road and bumped across the ground to get a closer look. The mustangs raised their heads and gazed at us, then galloped off, their coats glistening in the sunshine. Two young "long yearlings" (horses almost two years old) were full of curiosity—they ran bravely up close to us, then cut in front of our path before they took off at a dead run, carrying their tails gaily as if proud of their own courage.

I was touring the area at the request of the American Horse Protection Association, an organization I am active in. Because I'm a horse veterinarian, the association had asked for my opinion on the health and general condition of the mustangs here.

A big controversy was going on over the mustangs, and not for the first time. These noble animals have had to fight for survival—against the land, the climate, and often against people. In the past, they were at the mercy of anyone who came along, and local people regularly rounded them up and sold them for slaughter to the pet food companies. The horses were unprotected, peacefully grazing on public land, and it was just free fishing for the wranglers. In the 1920s and thirties, and even more recently, mustanging was a very profitable business. These roundups sometimes attracted public attention because of their unspeakable brutality. The terrified horses were driven off cliffs, hunted and herded by helicopters, clubbed, and disabled. Wranglers often put baling wire through the noses of unruly mustangs, tying down their nostrils so they could hardly breathe; when the horses were exhausted and half-smothered, they became easier to handle.

With enough evidence and documentation of what went on in mustanging, a Nevada woman, Mrs. Velma Johnston (Wild Horse Annie, she's called), fought the cause of the mustangs. Annie, a remarkable woman, has devoted her life to protecting these animals. Finally, with the help of conservationists and a large horse-loving public, she succeeded in getting Congress to pass a law making it illegal to hunt wild horses with aircraft. Later, a second law, the Wild Free-Roaming Horses and Burros Act of 1971, was passed, which gave somewhat more protection to these animals.

But though the horses can no longer legally be rounded up and sold for slaughter, the threat to them has not ended. I was in Nevada now to investigate another move to evict the mustangs. Four hundred were about to be rounded up because the Bureau of Land Management, BLM, a Department of Interior agency that has jurisdiction over the mustangs, was insisting that there were too many of them, and they were in danger of starvation. The BLM was planning to put the captured horses up for "adoption." Some had already been forced into corrals by the closing off of water holes in the valley. Three had already died. "Difficult" ones were to be tranquilized with dangerous drugs, or shot.

The big ranchers of the area were behind this roundup. These cattlemen are allowed to graze their cattle on the vast public lands. They pay no taxes on the land, of course, since it belongs to the government, and they pay only a token fee—about $1.60 per month per head—for grazing rights. (That is nothing compared to what a Midwestern or Eastern farmer has to pay to feed a cow!) I think it is all perfectly fine to put the land to use—but the ranchers say the horses compete with their cattle for forage. They seem to begrudge every blade of grass the mustangs eat. Now the ranchers were saying that forage was short, and the number of horses ought to be reduced—certainly not the number of their cattle. They had persuaded the BLM to remove half of this particular herd of mustangs. The BLM has consistently sought to get rid of all the mustangs in the West—by any method, including airborne roundups.

When I heard of all this from the American Horse Protection Association, I thought it was an outrage. In the first place, I was surprised to hear there wasn't enough food growing on the range. Wild horses require less forage than cattle. Over the centuries, the hardy mustangs have adapted far better than cattle to the scrubby grasses of the Western ranges. And indeed, those I had seen for myself since I got here looked in good condition—not at all emaciated.

Secondly, I could see no reason why the taxpayers

should pay to remove mustangs, which belong to all of us, just so the local big ranchers could get cheap grazing for their cattle. The roundup would cost five times more money than the grazing fees from the ranchers would bring in.

Mustangs are small horses, not very beautiful, and do not make good saddle horses. Who would "adopt" them? What would prevent their "adoptors" from selling them to the pet food companies?

There was even something funny about the number of horses the BLM said were in the herds in this part of Nevada. A few years earlier, the BLM had made a count and said there were some 450 horses in the area. Now, five years later, the figure has doubled! It takes eleven months for a mare to foal and one and a half years before young female horses go into heat. When I was there, I saw very few foals. In fact, there's no biological way a herd of 450 could become 900 in five years!

"How do you explain this sudden increase in your estimate?" I asked the BLM representative who was with us.

"Oh," said he, "we have better ways of counting the animals now."

It's true public lands are limited, so it's necessary and right that some control be exercised over them. When range managers determine the capacity of a given area of land, they figure it out scientifically in terms of AMUs—Animal Monthly Units. That's how many animals can be sustained in a normal month. In this area, the range managers had assigned a couple of thousand AMUs to wildlife, the rest to private cattle, and none to the horses.

One of the points our Horse Protection Organization has been pressing for is to get an agreement that a given amount of government land be reserved for the wild horses. It could be, say, one-fourth of the total of government land in the Western states where wild horses live. Then the agencies could realistically and accurately figure out if any wild horse herds had indeed exceeded the number that their allotted grazing space could comfortably sustain.

The mustangs are part of our country's heritage. They are harmful to no one and cost nothing to maintain. They have some protection now from those terrible abuses of the past; yet every few years a move is made to further harass, terrorize, injure, dispossess, and even kill them. Any ecologist familiar with animals knows that it is possible for wild animals to overbreed their territory, and perhaps some limited roundups are necessary, now and in the future. But I could see no reason for this one. And if future roundups are essential, I would like to see them planned responsibly by knowledgeable people with no self-interest involved, so that no harm will come to the animals.

I testified in court that the horses were not starving and were not reproducing rapidly. We were successful in making the BLM stop this roundup in Nevada temporarily and free the horses that had already been captured. But we lost in the end. It may soon be all over for the mustangs.

How did I become a horse veterinarian? Oddly enough, I was a city boy who'd never even heard of alfalfa hay until I was a junior in college! Though I was born in Nebraska, we moved to San Diego when I was nine. I think my interest in becoming a vet stems from my love for my constant boyhood companion, a Boston terrier named Murphy. I wanted Murphy to live as long as possible— and in fact, he did live to be fourteen years old.

During high school and part of college, I worked as a kennel boy in a small animal hospital and got my first experience with veterinary medicine—enough to know it was what I wanted. Then one summer I had a job assisting a racetrack veterinarian. I also worked as a relief milker in a dairy and as a general working hand on a cattle ranch. I became more and more fascinated by large animals. I got my degree in zoology at UCLA and went on to veterinary school at the University of California at Davis—finally, after having been turned down twice! I think my experiences working with animals helped as much as my grades in getting me admitted.

After I graduated from veterinary college, I worked for two years for a country veterinarian who had a mixed practice—about 80 percent dairy, 20 percent small animals. It was good experience.

Then twelve years ago I moved up here to Contra Costa County and began to specialize exclusively in horses. This area is ranch country. Do you know there are more horses per capita per square mile here than almost anywhere else in the United States—more even than around Lexington, Kentucky? There are five other horse veterinarians here, and we all keep busy. Most of our clients are youngsters who have their own horses for recreation. My patients are nearly all pleasure and show horses.

Equine veterinarians do about 60 percent of their work in the spring. It's not unusual to work twelve or fourteen hours a day during these months. That's the foaling season, also the breeding season because the mares come into heat then.

A great deal of my routine work is vaccinating and worming. We vaccinate for four main horse diseases—tetanus, influenza, equine encephalitis (sleeping sickness), and a respiratory disease called rhinopneumanitis. Horses are very prone to internal worms and should receive worm medicine every three months. Twice a year it's necessary to pass a tube through the horse's nose and down its throat and pump a mixture of worm medicine into its stomach. (Oddly enough, most horses take this procedure very well.) The rest of the time you can just put worm medicine in the grain. I usually worm and vaccinate my patients in groups—the youngsters bring their horses in on a Saturday, and I'll take care of twenty to fifty at a time.

Another kind of routine work I do is keeping my patients' teeth in good condition. The older horses especially need dental care. A horse's teeth continue to grow throughout its life, so they have to be filed down regularly to help it eat properly and prevent impaction (blockage of the intestine) from hay not chewed up well. This filing is called "floating"; I do it by hand, and it's hard work.

You've heard the expression "Put an old horse out to pasture." It's supposed to be an old horse's ideal reward for a lifetime of work. Well, the fact is, you should *never* put an old horse out to pasture! Just as old people require a great deal more attention and care, so do old horses. They get teeth trouble, stomach ailments, arthritis; their health problems increase. Many owners do not realize the pain a lame old horse is having. Some even believe it's normal for an old horse to be thin. This is not true; any older horse receiving good care has good general weight. If an owner can't give an old horse continual care, the humane thing is to have it put to sleep.

I can't describe the personal satisfaction I get out of being able to help animals when they need it. Even giving simple routine care—some of it is tremendously gratifying. Like examining the newborn foals. I get a lot of pleasure out of seeing the little babies struggle to their feet and begin to nurse for the first time. I wouldn't want to be in any other profession.

It was while I was the manager of a thoroughbred farm, before I started my own practice, that I formed some strong opinions about horse racing. I used to take care of some of our ranch horses at the track, so I got a good look at horse racing behind the scenes.

I am totally and completely opposed to racing two-year-olds. The bones of a young horse are not completely solid until it is nearly five years old. At two, the bones certainly aren't strong enough for the horse to be in racetrack competition. It's like putting a Little League kid into a major league ball game! Do you know that over 60 percent of two-year-old racehorses break down in their first year of racing?

It's the people who make the racing rules and set the purses who are responsible. Terrific pressure is put onto breeders to condition their horses to be ready at two years. I've seen trainers on the backs of twelve-month-old babies, forcing them to prepare for racing. If a horse doesn't win some races as a two-year-old, it's very hard for it to get a stall at a track as a three-year-old. I have no idea why the racing industry doesn't wait until the young horses are at least thirty months old—I guess it's the money involved. Racing is a multimillion-dollar industry. And yet, when so many of the two-year-olds are hurt and even ruined by racing, it hardly seems profitable for the owners.

Since all race horses born during any spring are considered to be one year old the following January first, even an eighteen-month-old horse may be forced to compete, and six months is a big difference in very young horses. If a little horse has the heart to run, it will often run beyond the capacity of its muscles to hold its legs together. Some even break their legs while running—the bones just snap.

The abuse of two-year-olds is compounded by the widespread use of a drug called Butazoladine, which is normally used to reduce inflammation and swelling. But Butazoladine is also a painkiller. Because it masks pain, a horse can extend itself beyond its physical capacity without realizing it. It's against the law to give a race horse a stimulant to make it run faster, or a tranquilizer to help control it during a race, but there's no law against the use of Butazoladine.

If people would only realize what really goes on in the racing of two-year-olds, maybe they would stop supporting it. The fans see the horses running, and they look beautiful, but the fans don't go into the barns later and see these poor animals in pain, with their legs all swollen and bandaged.

Another thing most people aren't aware of is the abuse of animals in rodeos. I have been a veterinarian at a cow palace, and at county fair rodeos. I've seen the injuries and pain the animals suffer.

I'm not talking about the bucking strap, the tight strap they buckle around a horse's lower abdomen, as he comes out of a chute, that makes him frantically uncomfortable —it presses on a tender area and drives him crazy, so he leaps and bucks trying to get it off. That's the least offensive thing at rodeos, if you want to make a priority list.

I mean the way a cowboy rakes a horse's shoulders with sharp spurs during the bronc-riding events, for one thing. The cowboy is trying to show how well he can maintain his balance on a bucking horse. But if he used rubber spurs, he could still show the action and not inflict excruciating pain on the horse.

Calf roping is another abuse. They force the animal out into the rodeo ring running full blast, then they rope it and jerk it right off its feet. You know how often you see the little roped calf dragged out of the ring, and the announcer says something about its having "got the wind knocked out of it"? The calf hasn't had the wind knocked out of it, its neck has been broken! A few years ago the University of Colorado veterinary school made a study and found by autopsies that many calves' necks are broken in rodeo calf roping. This could be avoided by using ropes with a stretch section in them or by following the rules that apply to some women's events—once the calf is roped, the rope is simply released without making the calf bite the dust.

I realize that rodeos are a big Western tradition, and I'm not putting down the whole rodeo business. Some rodeo participants do it right, without causing the animals to suffer. But most don't bother. I believe all the participants could develop the same riding and roping skills in a humane way and still keep the thrill in rodeos.

Perhaps the most outright cruelty inflicted on the horse today is the soring of the Tennessee Walking Horses. These horses are a beautiful breed with a lot to offer. They have a unique, natural gait—a running walk that is so smooth you think you're riding on a cloud. In competition, these horses have a flashy action with their front feet that's called the Big Lick. They pick their feet up high in an exaggerated way.

The origin of soring is said to go back to a certain famous Walking Horse, Merry Go Boy, who had such an elegant action with his front feet that no other horse could compete with him. He was winning all the prizes. Because it's difficult to train a horse to show off this way, some trainers began to resort to soring as a way to make their horses look as good. Soring means using something artificial to purposely cause pain in a horse's front legs. Oil of mustard rubbed into the skin of a horse's heels will do it, or tight chains, or bell-like collars put around the foot. People have used all kinds of vicious methods to hurt the horses' front feet so they will walk with most of their weight on the back legs and lift the sore feet high. The trainers and judges and the audiences think this looks great, but the sored horses are in agony.

One of the reasons the American Horse Protection Association came into being was to stop the practice of soring. The founders of the organization brought publicity to bear and were instrumental in getting the Horse Protection Act of 1970 passed, which outlaws soring. But as often happens, getting the law enforced is another matter.

Because I'm a horse veterinarian, the association asked me to go to Shelbyville, Tennessee, to the big National Walking Horse Celebration to see if the law was being observed and enforced and report to Congress about it.

Well, I had heard the practice of soring was bad, but I had had no firsthand experience with it. I'd seen pictures, but had never seen what a sored horse really looks like. I'll never forget it.

I went around to the horses' stalls before and after the events. Many of the horses were lying down because they couldn't stand. Some were moaning. Many even lay down to eat, which no healthy horse ever does. The trainers would force them to their feet and prod them into the show ring with sticks. Some horses had been sored so much that the tissues of their legs had become like parchment paper and bled easily. You'd see blood running down their pasterns as they came from the show ring. I've seen a lot of abuses to animals in the course of my life, but this was one of the worst.

After the authorities began to crack down, the Tennessee Walking Horse breeders and trainers became more sophisticated and now don't sore their horses in such an obvious way. They do things like inject iodine under the skin of the horses' legs. There's no injury that can actually be seen, but the tissues of the leg become severely irritated. Now, an irritated area will be hot. Fortunately, an instrument has been developed in recent years that picks up extra heat in a horse's legs and will register if an irritant has been used.

The Department of Agriculture veterinarians, who are now in charge of enforcing the Horse Protection Act, catch some instances of soring with this device.

Of course, not all breeders and trainers want to sore their horses. Many would never resort to it if it weren't for the others who do. But their horses have to compete with the high-stepping horses that have been sored. There's big money involved, so the decent people feel they are forced into soring.

One day several years ago, a family drove up to my house with an injured fawn. Their teenage son was holding it in his arms.

"We found it on the road," the woman said. "It had been hit by a car and was just lying there helpless."

"So we picked it up and took it to the nearest filling station, where we phoned the Fish and Game office to ask what to do with it," her husband said. "You know what they told us? We should either leave it alone or dispose of it—if we didn't want to do it ourselves, we could bring it to them and they would do the job for us. Why should this animal be killed if it has a chance to recover? It has a right to live."

"Bring it in and let me have a look at it," I said.

I examined the baby deer and saw that it had a concussion and some bad lacerations and bruises, but fortunately no broken bones.

"I think its injuries will heal up nicely," I said. "Do you have a place where you can care for it while it recovers?"

The people lived in the city and couldn't very well keep it themselves. The upshot was they left it with me. I took care of it and raised it. It grew to be a beautiful young doe, and when she was old enough, I released her up in the mountains.

But the incident made me realize there was no formal setup to take care of injured wildlife. I checked around—talked to the Fish and Game office and the Humane Society and found out that people were continually calling them, asking what to do with injured wild animals they had found.

It seemed to me this was an area that veterinarians might become involved in. A lot of vets I know are concerned about wildlife. So I contacted an attorney and, with the help of some local people, formed what we call the National Wildlife Health Foundation. Now almost 250 veterinarians all over the country are on our roster of "Active Wildlife Veterinarians." They make themselves known through local humane societies and animal-control agencies.

Remember when those big offshore oil spills occurred a few years back, and everybody was out trying to clean the oil off the wild seabirds? After the first spill, I called the Fish and Game people and asked if they wanted any help. They said they'd be glad to have a veterinarian involved, so I went down and got permission to bring back about ninety birds. We had cages all over my kitchen and enclosed patio.

A big problem soon became evident to everybody trying to help these birds. The detergents that people used for cleaning the crude oil off the birds' feathers also removed the natural oils that made their feathers waterproof. When their feathers got wet, the birds died. Only about 5 percent of the birds survived after being cleaned of crude oil.

Two years later there was a second big oil calamity—two tankers collided, and about 5,000 birds got drenched in oil. This time we tried using light mineral oil instead of detergent to clean the feathers. It worked better, but we still lost a large percentage of the birds.

However, after this incident our foundation got a grant from the Standard Oil Company to work on the problem. A biochemist, Dr. Allen G. Pittman, and I started doing research to find the right kind of solvent. He discovered that detergents left a microscopic film on the birds' feathers that attracted water, which in turn killed the birds. We knew of fluids that would remove the crude oil without leaving a film, but those would be toxic if the birds absorbed them through their skin. Finally we found a solvent that works and is safe—Shell Sol 70, it's called. Birds will be waterproof and can go back to the wild within three days of being cleaned with it. I wrote a manual about it— "After-Care of Oil-Covered Birds"—which our foundation published.

Is it safe for people to pick up sick or injured wildlife? I think the answer is yes and no. Some injured animals might bite because they're in pain; you have to be very careful. Clearly a bird caught in an oil slick or a deer that has obviously been hit by a car is not dangerous to handle. But a small animal acting *sick* is another matter because of the danger of rabies. Sick foxes, raccoons, squirrels, and skunks should be approached with extreme caution. We discourage people from handling any wild animal that seems ill rather than injured. We advise them to get an experienced animal patrol or Humane Society officer to capture it and bring it to one of our vets.

I find myself coming out strongly against so many things involving animals, I suppose I may sound fanatic to some people. But as a veterinarian, I know animals, and whenever I have to defend my position, I find I'm on very firm ground.

If you really care about animals, I think you have to

examine the activities and institutions concerning them. You have to stand back and think, Is this really right?

When I was a kid, an uncle used to take me pheasant hunting. I thought it was great, getting up early in the morning, going out in the woods, watching my uncle's Labrador go on point. It seemed very exciting to me at the time. I didn't really understand what I was doing until years later, after I had actually graduated from veterinary school. One day I was hunting, and I shot a bird close to me and completely demolished it. I picked up what was left of that beautiful bird—a head and some feathers—and suddenly thought, What in the world am I doing? I suddenly saw myself, the hunter, from the bird's point of view. I also saw myself as somebody getting his kicks by killing a harmless living thing. That was the last time I touched a gun.

Perhaps some very poor people truly need to hunt to feed themselves and their families. And I realize that a few people (very few) are expert shots and are able to kill an animal instantly every time. But most hunters are there for the pleasure they get out of hunting, and they inflict cruelty without a second thought. (Bow-and-arrow hunters, they're the worst; they cause more suffering than anyone else. I've seen so many injured animals and even birds with arrows stuck in them.) And what kind of skill or bravery does it require to let a pack of dogs chase a mountain lion up a tree, where it can't get away, and then shoot it from a distance of a few feet?

People say they like hunting because it gives them a chance to be out in the woods away from the rat race, or it gives them an opportunity to have a man-to-man relationship with their sons. They are kidding themselves. They could do all the other outdoor things—hike, camp out in the woods, study nature and wildlife, climb mountains, go canoeing, whatever—if that were what they *really* wanted. If their interest were marksmanship, they could shoot at targets.

Some people who don't defend hunting as a sport nevertheless say it is necessary. They claim that because there is more wildlife than our wildernesses can support, it is kinder to shoot down animals than to let them die slowly from starvation.

Well, one reason why we have an excessive number of wild animals in many places is that through wildlife management the state Fish and Game people purposely improve the habitat of *huntable* animals—just so there will be too many each year, and hunters can be assured of animals to kill. By manipulating the environment—eliminating the natural predators, or burning out overgrown brush, for example—wildlife management encourages certain animals to overbreed (by no coincidence, animals that hunters like to hunt). The original intention of wildlife management was to prevent overpopulation or overhunting of one of our natural resources—wildlife. Now, the system has become merely a tool of the hunting and fishing organizations. In most instances, the overpopulation of huntable animals is an artificially created situation.

The subject of hunting brings me to another popular institution that I feel inflicts great cruelty on animals—the zoo. As far as I'm concerned, zoos should be eliminated.

I really feel that wild animals should be allowed to live exclusively in their natural habitat. I am perfectly aware that man has changed the world greatly, and that the spread of civilization has made it increasingly impossible for many wild animals to exist. But I am opposed to putting them in prisons. You have seen caged animals pacing, walking in circles, shaking their heads back and forth. That's caused by the stress and boredom of captivity. I think they would be better off dead.

In the first place, the capturing of animals to meet the demands of zoos, laboratories, and exotic pet suppliers is both cruel and irresponsible. For every single rare animal that lives to be sold, as many as a dozen have died during capture, or being held for transport, or being transported. The capture and shipment of apes and monkeys is an especially wretched business. The traditional way to obtain one is to kill a mother and take her baby. If the infant isn't killed in the fall from the trees when the mother is shot, its chances of surviving the capture, the time spent in the holding area, the shipment, and the stay at the animal dealer's are still poor. Jane Goodall, the expert on chimpanzees who spent many years studying them in Africa, estimates that for every live baby chimp who arrives in Europe or the United States, six have lost their lives.

Some zoo curators and directors justify the existence of zoos by saying that they preserve species that are becoming extinct. But in many cases wild animal populations have actually been reduced in their home environments because the hunters and dealers can make money selling the creatures. Zoos are a market for the animals, and as such, tend to deplete some of the animal species they claim they are preserving.

The indifferent treatment and even abuse many zoo animals suffer is another reason to question the wisdom and morality of having zoos at all. If the word "prison" seems strong, I call your attention to the case of Ziggy, an elephant at a zoo in Illinois who was kept in solitary confinement, literally chained in a dungeon cellar for thirty years, because once during his mating season he had become unruly and attacked his trainer. The elephant had apparently been "sentenced" to the dungeon as punishment and forgotten until somebody discovered him years later and raised a public fuss. Finally the zoo unchained him and moved him to quarters aboveground. Ziggy was weak and nearly blind by then, of course. This may be an unusual and extreme case, but it illustrates the type of thinking that can be involved in zoo keeping.

I once heard the pathologist of the San Diego Zoo, one of the best zoos in the world, lecture on causes of death among zoo animals, and do you know what he named as a major killer? Malnutrition. We've been keeping animals in zoos for hundreds, perhaps thousands, of years and still don't know how to feed them properly.

Large natural wildlife refuges are something different. I don't mean those little safarilands—people think of them as vast acreages, but actually there isn't enough room for the animals to live without killing each other off. A really big natural game refuge is something else.

It's hard to be against what most people take for granted, but I think all zoos should be phased out. What I'd like to see instead are wildlife study centers in every community. A good natural history museum with dioramas and good visual aids can teach a lot more about the real nature of animals than any zoo. Looking at some poor arthritic lion pacing miserably in a concrete cage tells you very little about this interesting beast. A good museum with wildlife films, slide shows, earphones with commentary explaining the dioramas—that's the really educational and beneficial way to enjoy wildlife. The natural history museums in San Diego and New York are wonderful examples.

I saw a children's toy the other day that struck me as an example of how animal abuse is taken for granted. This toy consists of a plastic truck with a large net attached and a plastic rhinoceros. The child plays with the toy by using the truck and net to capture the animal. The message the child gets is that wildlife is something to be hunted, captured, and/or killed, not something to be appreciated and conserved in its natural habitat. This is how kids learn the values of our culture. Once this view is engendered, it's hard to change it.

I'd like to see everybody happy—people and animals. We are all sharing this planet. But as things are now, the majority of animals are getting a raw deal. So many abuses are the norm within our culture, that it's difficult to convince people there's anything wrong. Most people are not intentionally cruel, they are simply unaware.

Animal lovers and decent people who want to end animal abuse have to question the institutions and practices we all take for granted. We have to ask, What's happening to the animals? And if it's not good, we have to do something about it.

7. "Cats are special, and people who own cats know that."

Cats seem to go on the principle that it never does any harm to ask for what you want.

—JOSEPH WOOD KRUTCH

New York City not only has a huge human population—it also has one of the largest concentrations of pets in the world. There are dogs, cats, birds, mice, fish, snakes—even exotic pets such as monkeys. A veterinarian can earn a living specializing exclusively in his or her favorite small animal—and that's what Kathy Atamian has done.

Two years ago, young Dr. Atamian took the plunge, rented a loft in Greenwich Village, and opened up her own cat hospital. With the help of some friends who were competent handypersons, she partitioned the loft space into a waiting room, an office, an examining room, a surgery, patient quarters, and storage. She was able to borrow money for her equipment. Today she and her helpers, cat lovers all, have come through the ups and downs of these first years and (like cats) landed on their feet.

The Midwest veterinary school I went to was very large-animal oriented. We had two weeks of lectures on farm animals for every hour devoted to small animals. I used to wonder when I would ever get a chance to take care of cats.

But after graduation, I came east and worked for three years at the Animal Medical Center in New York, first as an intern and then as a resident. Interns and residents are graduate doctors selected to work under supervision at a teaching hospital. Both experiences are valuable training, although not required for practice. I certainly saw plenty of dogs and cats at the AMC—and I think I saw more unusual cases than I'll probably come across in fifteen years of practice, even in New York. And the center is so well-equipped and has such a remarkable bunch of people that I got used to having the best of everything.

I decided to stay in New York, and when I finished my residency, I spent another two years working for Dr. John Levy, an established veterinarian with a busy practice. Finally I thought I was ready, so I got up the nerve to go on my own.

When I announced I wanted to open a practice devoted exclusively to cats, most of the people I knew had negative reactions.

"You'll go broke," said a colleague. "It's not like specializing in horses, out in the country, where most of your work is done in your clients' barns. You'll need a clinic, costly equipment; you won't get enough patients to cover your high expenses, especially in an inflation-ridden city like New York."

"It will be hard to turn away people who walk in with their dogs," commented Dr. Levy, my former employer.

"Just cats!" exclaimed my brother-in-law. "People will think you're nuts."

But cats are special, I explained, and people who own

cats know that. It will make perfectly good sense to most cat owners when they hear I treat only cats. I believe that cats are so different from all other animals, so subtle and interesting, that I could fill a lifetime just learning new things about them.

A friend painted a little sign for me that said "K. Atamian, D.V.M.," with a picture of a cat, and I hung it downstairs by the bell to my clinic.

One morning a few weeks after I had opened for business, a woman rushed in with a carrying case.

"My cat fell out of a sixth-story window!" she said urgently. "I don't have an appointment, I just picked him up and dashed over, hoping you'd be here, Doctor." And she showed me her cat.

I had seen many, many similar cases when I was at the Animal Medical Center and also at Dr. Levy's and had assisted at dozens of orthopedic operations for setting broken bones. People have the notion that cats don't fall out of windows. One single day spent at any busy small-animal hospital would change their minds. Every spring, I get one or two window cases *a day* myself. Cats rarely fall out of trees because they can cling to tree bark with their claws; but they can't dig their claws into concrete or brick. They fall out of windows all the time, killing or injuring themselves. We call it the "high-rise syndrome." Owners should protect their cats from this.

"We *never* open our windows from the bottom unless the screens are securely in place," said this woman, as if she were reading my mind. "We have several cats; we know about cats and windows. But my son had a friend over, the two of them were in his room, and I guess Steve didn't notice that his friend opened the window behind the venetian blind." She lifted her cat gently from the carrying case and placed him on my examining table.

"Poor kitty," I said. "Let's have a look at you."

The cat, a young gray male, crouched miserably on the table and growled as I touched him.

"I think his left hind leg is broken," said his owner. "I can't believe that's all, though—six stories down to the sidewalk!"

My assistant, Paul, held the cat firmly on the table while I examined him. The common procedure in examining a cat is stem to stern—start with the head and work your way along the body toward the rear. This cat's nose was a little bloody, but from a superficial wound, not a nosebleed. I decided he had simply scraped his nose when he'd hit the sidewalk. I felt his chest and abdomen; nothing seemed to be wrong. His heartbeat and respiration were somewhat elevated, but this was not unusual for a cat who has had such a fall. His front legs moved easily, were not swollen, and did not seem to hurt him. Then I got to the hind legs.

Meanwhile Janet, my receptionist, was taking the cat's history from the owner, a Mrs. Welles. Fred, as this cat was called, was two years old and in good health, alert and lively, with a glossy coat. He was a little shy, Mrs. Welles said, but devoted to the members of his family.

Fred had a broken hind leg, all right—but how badly broken I couldn't tell. I gave him a sedative and an injection of antibiotics.

"I'll have to X-ray his leg," I said to Mrs. Welles, "and then set it and put a cast on it. Also, Fred should stay here at least overnight so we can keep an eye on him to be sure he doesn't develop any other complications." I reassured her as best I could; she was understandably upset about her pet.

As soon as the sedative had made Fred more relaxed, Paul and I took X rays of his leg. It was a T-shaped fracture, one of the worst kinds. I had seen a few somewhat like it, and they are difficult to repair because the bones have to knit back together three ways. I had assisted at similar orthopedic operations, and I knew how to do it. Still, I had a pang of nervousness; was I being overconfident in attempting it myself?

We put Fred under anesthesia and I operated on the leg. Setting it was some delicate job; I had a lot of trouble getting the bone fragments to align correctly. I put in a bone screw and several metal pins to hold the break together, and then put on a cast. To tell the truth, it would have been a fancy piece of surgery even for some of the big shots I had assisted at the Animal Medical Center. I felt I had succeeded.

Fred was able to go home two days later. One thing about cats and dogs—they always forgive their owners for taking them to the hospital in the first place when their owners come to take them back home. You could hear Fred purr all the way out the door in his carrier.

But two weeks later, when he came back for a checkup, Fred looked more miserable than ever. The X ray revealed that the pins had not held, and the bones had slipped out of alignment. I showed the X ray to Mrs. Welles.

"I can see what you mean. The bones aren't right—this one is sticking up where it obviously shouldn't," she said. "I guess this means you'll have to operate over again?"

"Yes. I'll have to put in several more pins, and this time I'll also wire the bones together. He'll be able to walk, although that leg may always be stiff."

I wondered if Mrs. Welles thought I was incompetent. I wondered if she would take Fred elsewhere rather than let me do the second operation. I wondered if she would think my bill exorbitant if I charged her what would be a fair fee for the surgery and care. I only hope I didn't show my anxiety. Oh, Dr. Levy, why did I ever think I wanted my own practice?

So far in my practice, I had been very lucky. At that time, I had already done maybe thirty spays and castrations, treated a number of urinary obstructions, upper respiratory infections, and a skin allergy successfully. I'd removed a benign tumor with no complications. I hadn't lost a cat yet, not even several who were brought to me almost too late to treat. I hoped Fred's case wasn't going to be my first failure.

I *could* chicken out with Fred and recommend that Mrs. Welles take him up to the center. But that would be admitting that I wasn't brave enough to do my very best at what I had been trained to do. After all, I told myself, my former boss and the teachers at the center had not always succeeded the first time with every orthopedic case.

I had one thing going for me—Fred was a healthy cat with a great spirit and will to recover. He bore his cast with dignity. He was greatly loved by his owners (a big factor in a pet's recovery chances).

Mrs. Welles told me to go ahead and do what I thought was necessary. She didn't faint when I told her what my bill would be—she only asked if she could pay it off in several installments. I agreed gratefully. Sometimes you take a chance on never getting your money, but I trusted this lady.

I wish I could tell you that I operated on Fred successfully and he went home and lived happily ever after. But about a week after Fred had gone home the second time, Mrs. Welles phoned and said that something was wrong. Fred had been eating normally and moving about quite well with his cast—was even able to jump into a chair with it—but for several days now he had been lying under a bed, wouldn't move, and seemed terribly depressed.

"Better bring him right in," I said with a sinking heart. Mrs. Welles came in with Fred about an hour later.

Paul and I cut the cast off. This time it wasn't the surgery that had gone wrong—it was a much simpler problem, thank goodness. The cast had been pressing on Fred's leg joint and had worn a bad sore there that hurt the poor cat when he walked. That's why he wouldn't move from the spot under the bed. I will never get over my distress that an animal can't tell you when or where something hurts. This time I left the cast off so the sore could heal, and put Fred in one of my cages, rather than let him go home, where he would move about.

When I set up my clinic here, I insisted on homelike, cozy cages for my in-patients. I vowed I would never have those cold, steel cages I had seen in most animal hospitals. My cages are wood, with pillows for the patients to lie on, a little shelf halfway up in one corner where they can sit if they like, a clean litter pan, and a bowl of water at all times. Sure, some of the cats knock over the water bowl, or lie in the litter pan, or vomit on the pillow. My cages are a lot of work, but I believe it is worth it for my patients. We put Fred in a quiet one at the back of the clinic.

One of my assistants spent time each day holding Fred and petting him. I provide this extra nursing care for all my patients. Every day an assistant takes each patient on her lap and strokes and talks to it for at least twenty minutes. I think this often gives a sick cat the will to live. A cat left alone in a cage, homesick as well as ill or injured, never handled except to have medication thrust down its throat or a needle stuck in it or a bandage changed—why shouldn't the cat just give up?

This kind of care seemed to help Fred. After ten days or so, the sore on his leg healed, and he went home. He came back for checkups, improved steadily, and regained almost full use of his leg.

Fred is still my patient; Mrs. Welles brought him in the other day for his yearly distemper shot. Fred is a fine, healthy cat. I questioned his owner about the use of his leg.

"He can hop, skip, and jump as well as ever," she told me. "The only thing he can't do is tuck the leg under him properly when he sits. It sticks out in front of him a bit. It looks a little funny, but Fred doesn't seem to notice."

Fred's stiff leg reminded me of a story my father had once told me about a dog he had on his Colorado farm when he was a boy. This dog had broken a hind leg somehow; it had been set by the local veterinarian, and while it was healing, the dog ran about on three legs, holding the injured one up. My Dad said the dog got so used to running on three legs that he did it the rest of his life. The only thing was, the dog forgot which leg had been broken —so sometimes he held his left leg up, and sometimes his right! I wonder if a cat would be so muddle-headed. I once read an essay called "Notes on Cathood" by Alastair Reid, in which he says something to the effect that dogs think, but cats know. I'm inclined to believe it. Wise with a sort of understanding human beings cannot measure, cats function on something more than cerebral activity.

The problem of strays that people bring in is much harder for me to handle than difficult surgery cases such as Fred's. The city is swarming with abandoned and homeless cats, thanks to all the cat owners who do not have their cats altered. There are six cats who live at my clinic that I have simply never been able to find homes for. I acquired them from people who brought them in and then just never came back to pick them up. In fact, Kismet, my black cat, was dumped unceremoniously one morning by somebody who walked into the waiting room, set the cat on the floor, and fled. Poor Kismet was skin and bones, with three different kinds of parasites, a respiratory infection, and ulcers in her mouth. That was one time I was tempted to perform a mercy killing by giving an overdose of anesthetic. I didn't have the heart. Today, she is a magnificent cat, affectionate toward people, but not fond of other cats.

Some cats that have had to fend for themselves on the city streets make marvelous house pets, but others never get over their early experiences. A cat that has had to fight other cats for every mouthful of food to stay alive may take years to adjust to living peacefully with other cats. On the other hand, a cat who has been abused and terrorized by human beings may get along with its own kind but remain afraid of people; usually such a cat will eventually learn to trust its owner but will shy away from strangers.

People who abandon cats on the street are not always consciously cruel, they are simply lacking in awareness and empathy. They may actually believe they are doing the animal a favor by "giving it its freedom." The truth is that most abandoned cats die quite quickly and horribly from disease; they become undernourished and loaded with parasites. A kitten can be almost literally eaten alive by fleas. In their weakened condition, strays easily contract diseases—in the winter many develop pneumonia from exposure. If they are unaltered, the males fight and get infected wounds, while the females bear endless kittens, who in turn starve and die. Homeless cats get killed by cars, or are tortured by vicious people—you'd be amazed at the bizarre sadism cats are sometimes subjected to.

Occasionally, rarely, you see an exceptional street cat. Last winter one of my clients brought in a battle-scarred, good-natured old male cat, Muffin, who had lived in her neighborhood for years, fed by the neighbors and surviving by a lot of extraordinary good luck. My client had let him in her house because he seemed sick and the weather was icy. Muffin was sick all right—he had feline leukemia, and I could do nothing for him. Because feline leukemia is contagious, my client persuaded a friend who had no cat to take Muffin, so at least he died comfortably in a nice warm house where he was fed and petted to the end.

One of our resident cats, Gloria, was literally left on our doorstep. A woman telephoned, gave a name and address, and made an appointment. The doorbell rang at the time she was due, and she announced herself through the intercom. We were puzzled when nobody came up the stairs, but the office was busy, and we didn't think much about it. A little later, another patient came up and said there was a box on the sidewalk near the front door. Sure enough, we found a cat in it, a full-grown tortoiseshell, very pretty.

At first we thought she was seriously sick, because she just lay still, with her head in the corner of the box, showed no interest in her surroundings and didn't even look at us. After office hours, I examined her, and there was no sign of physical illness at all. The cat was simply despondent at being abandoned. She would not eat for over a week, just lay in her cage. I have never seen a cat so depressed. Finally, after steady care and coaxing, she came around. I am convinced she wouldn't have lasted two weeks on the street; she had no will to live at all and would have let herself die.

I must tell you about Mr. Mulvaney, one of our very special clients. You know how people who go around feeding stray cats are always depicted as weird little old ladies with shopping bags, recluse types who love cats but hate people? It's just not true. In my practice, I see all different kinds of people who love cats and feed strays. Mr. Mulvaney is certainly not somebody you would think of as eccentric. He is the managing editor of a big national magazine, as personable a guy as you're likely to meet. He lives in the suburbs with his wife and children and their own household of pet cats. Then he has some ten to twenty other cats that he has picked up and persuaded other people to keep temporarily for him.

Mr. Mulvaney has created a whole network of cat feeding stations all over New York City. These are vacant lots and empty buildings—places homeless cats congregate. Because he can't get to all his feeding stations on his lunch hour, he supplies food and has other people—volunteers—who fill in for him. You might say he manages the stray-cat situation for a large part of the city!

In addition, whenever he finds a cat that needs medical attention, Mr. Mulvaney captures it and brings it to me. I always have two or three of his cats convalescing at my place at any given time. I supply veterinary care and neutering to Mr. Mulvaney's cats free of charge, but this is a secret, because if it were widely known, I would have a hundred charity cats brought to me every day.

One of our favorite resident cats, Gina, was found by Mr. Mulvaney with a crushed leg; apparently she had been hit by a car. She was so sweet and trusting that she must have been recently abandoned. It was a Friday, a busy day for me; I operated on her after hours, at about eleven at night. Even in her pain, Gina was so affectionate that she would purr if you so much as looked at her. After a few days we let her out of the nook where we keep "family" cats when they're sick. "Family" means cats of my employees, cats who live here, my own personal cats, and Mr. Mulvaney's (he is considered "Family"). Gina hobbled around with an enormous heavy cast on her leg, purring among the clients and generally endearing herself to everybody. She quickly learned how to get people to help her. She would sit and look at a chair she wanted to sit in, or a door she wanted opened for her, and then when someone walked by, she would give this sweet little mew and look up at you. We'd all melt, no matter how busy we were.

Then after a couple of months, her leg was well, and we took the cast off. There was this skinny little leg, like a chicken leg! Apparently Gina was horrified. She limped for several weeks and wouldn't let anybody touch it. This angelic cat, who had been the darling of the place, became crotchety and cross, and growled if you tried to pet her. Then, perhaps too hastily, we found a home for her in a house where there was another pet cat. The owner was away all day and wanted another cat to keep her pet company so it wouldn't be lonely. Gina was chosen.

After a few weeks, the new owner called up and asked if we would take Gina back. Gina didn't like the other cat, wouldn't make friends with the new owner or anybody else. So she's back with us, as one of our resident cats, permanently, I guess. Now she is beginning to act more like her former sweet self. We sent another of Mr. Mulvaney's cats to be a companion to the other cat, and that worked out well.

I'm so fascinated by my pet cats and patients that I could go on and on telling stories about them. Sometimes my friends think I am too involved with my work because I put in such long hours—fifty to sixty hours a week. My boy friend complains, but fortunately he is in law school and very busy himself. One thing a would-be veterinarian has to consider is the dedication and sometimes the loneliness of the first years in practice. Perhaps eventually I will have a partner, so I can take a vacation and have more time to myself. I'll have to make some compromises, also, if I have a family, but I could never give up my work completely—it's far too interesting and fulfilling.

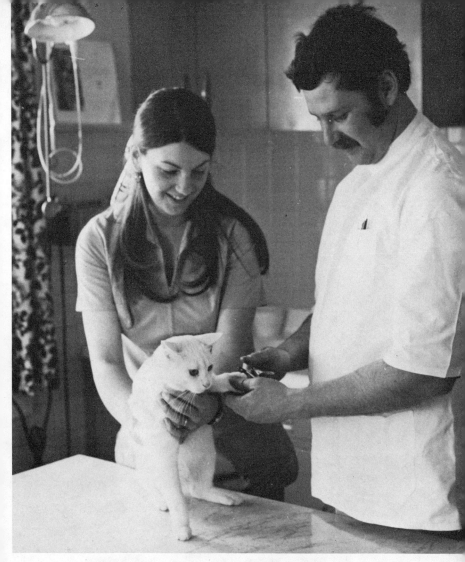

A veterinarian and his assistant examine a cat whose owners have consulted him about declawing because she is ruining an upholstered chair. Veterinarians differ in their opinion of declawing. "I am against it," says this small-animal practitioner. "Although we declaw only the front paws, the operation is very painful and often changes a cat's personality. Also, any cat might need its claws someday to defend itself or get up a tree to safety. The hind claws alone are not adequate for either need. I am recommending that instead of declawing the cat, the owners keep her claws blunt by trimming them regularly—then she can't damage their furniture." *Photo by Wendy Palitz.*

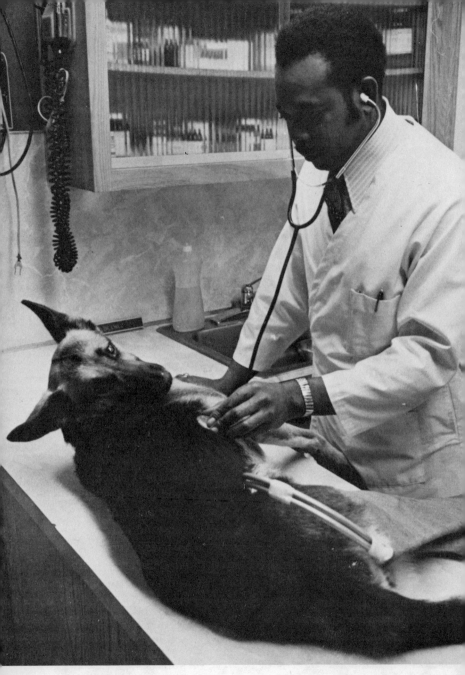

A veterinarian examines a German shepherd who was hit by a car and suffered a broken leg. He has set it in a special splint called a Thomas splint. "The dog is recovering nicely," says the vet. "I think I can let her go home tomorrow." *Photo by Dan Miller.*

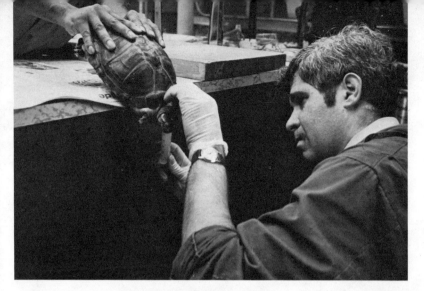

"One of our turtles is sick—he's been swimming in a corkscrew pattern and seems sluggish," says this zoo veterinarian. "I've discovered fluid in his body cavity, so I'm drawing some out to send to the lab for analysis. When we find out what's wrong, we can treat him." *Photo by Dan Miller.*

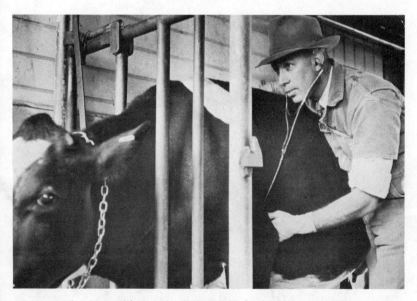

A large-animal practitioner checks out a Holstein dairy cow. "The farmer called me because she's been coughing," he says. "I'm listening to her lungs—we want to make sure she doesn't have pneumonia." *Photo by Joe Munroe, Photo Researchers, Inc.*

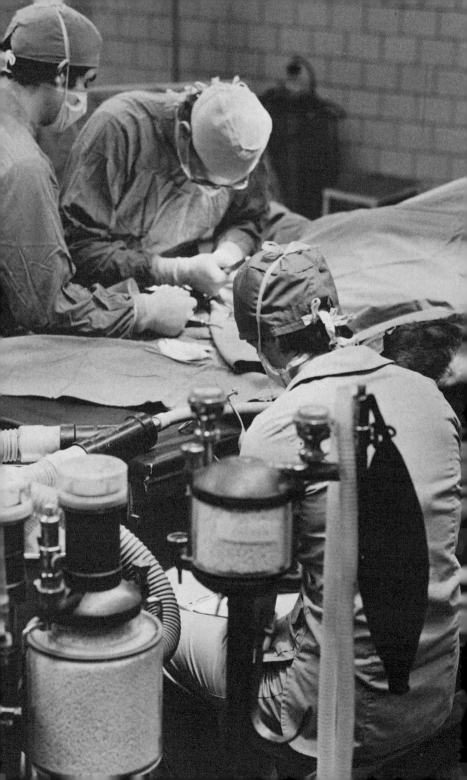

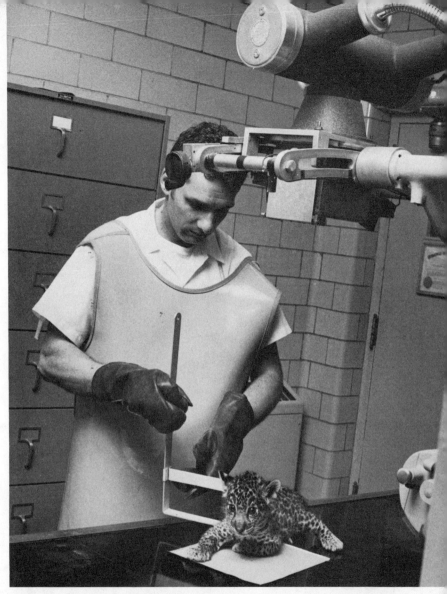

A jaguar kitten, pride and joy of a large zoo, has had a fall and seems to have hurt her leg. An animal technologist is taking X rays of the little animal's leg. "Our zoo vet is concerned that it might be fractured," he says. *Photo by Tom McHugh, Photo Researchers, Inc.*

(*left*) A surgical operation is in progress on a six-month-old colt whose front leg has grown crooked. "Two of my students are assisting me in placing a staple in the leg, which will help to straighten it as the horse continues to grow," explains the surgeon, a college professor. "Jeanne is administering the anesthesia, while David stands next to me and hands me the instruments." *Photo by Sol Goldberg, courtesy of Cornell University.*

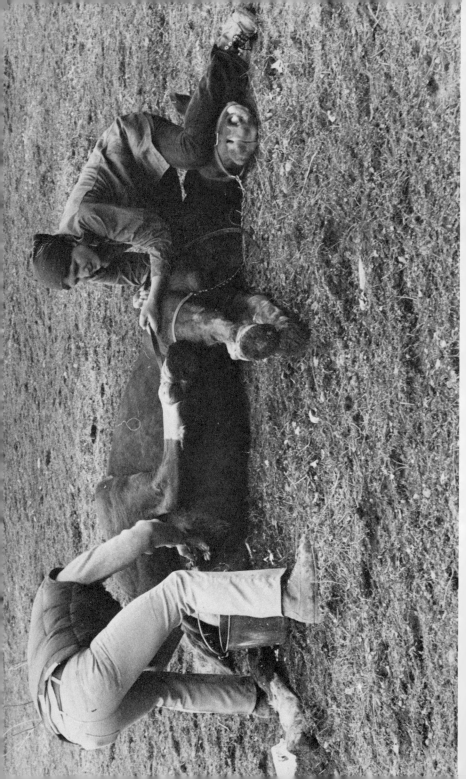

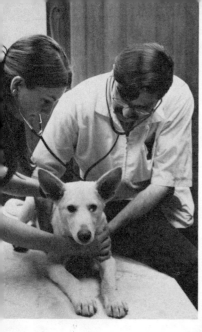

(*left*) A veterinary student and her professor listen to a young dog's heartbeat with a two-headed stethoscope, a teaching instrument that enables student and instructor to hear the same thing simultaneously. "The dog needs an operation to correct a serious heart defect called a patent ductus arteriosus," the professor says. "We expect he'll come through with flying colors and be able to live a normal life." *Photo by Wendy Palitz.*

(*right*) A zoo veterinarian gives an injection of antibiotics to a pony who has a mild respiratory infection. "I'm giving antibiotics to the whole herd," he explains, "to prevent anything more serious from developing." *Photo by Dan Miller.*

(*opposite*) A country practitioner gelds (castrates) a young horse. The operation is relatively simple, so he performs it right in the pasture. The horse has been given a complete anesthesia that is quite short-acting, so the veterinarian works quickly. His assistant holds the horse's foot up out of the way and sits on his head in case the horse should suddenly try to rise. "He'll be on his feet in a few minutes, puzzled but not too uncomfortable," comments the veterinarian. "This procedure should make him a more gentle pleasure horse." *Photo by Linda M. Salwen.*

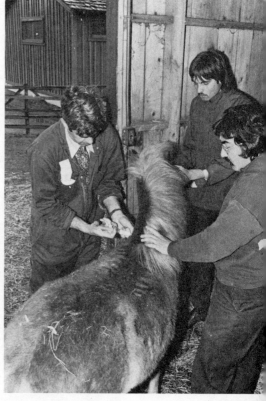

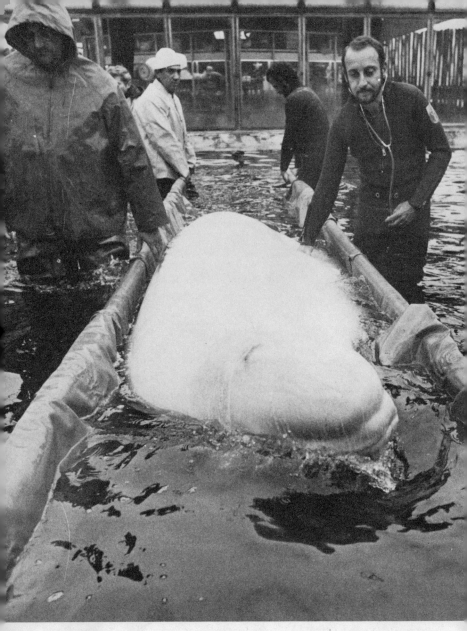

A marine mammal veterinarian has put on a "wet suit" and gotten into the tank to examine a female white whale at the aquarium where he is a consultant. "We're all excited because she is pregnant, and we are hoping she will successfully deliver a calf—a rare event," he comments. *Photo by Barton Silverman/NYT Pictures.*

8. "You've got to respect both the littlest dog and the biggest elephant."

Giraffes are without doubt the most spectacularly improbable of mammals.

—JULIAN HUXLEY

J. Y. Henderson has been the veterinarian for Ringling Bros. Barnum & Bailey Circus for thirty-four years, and no book on veterinarians would be complete without him. His job is rare in veterinary medicine. Some two-hundred performing animals—the good-natured elephants who lumber slow motion through their absurd antics, the magnificent big cats, the graceful horses, the comic little dogs—are under his watchful eye, both on tour and at the circus's winter quarters in Florida. In addition, Dr. Henderson is attending physician to the exotic animals of the sideshow, the Circus World Showcase, and other properties of Ringling.

A wiry, straight-as-an-arrow Texan, Doc Henderson likes to talk about his work—once even wrote a book about it, called *Circus Doctor*. Here, he tells a few anecdotes about his life with the Greatest Show on Earth.

One day when we were setting up the sideshow in a large city, the men unloaded the apes and monkeys in their cages and put them in temporary positions side by side, right up next to each other. We had a very friendly young orangutan named Floyd in a cage by himself. An orangutan is a red-haired ape about the size of a chimpanzee. Floyd got lonesome, I guess, or curious, or was just trying to make friends, but for whatever reason, he stuck his hand through the bars of the cage of a chimpanzee next to him.

Well, that poor orangutan got a nasty shock—the chimp grabbed his wrist and held it and went to work on the orangutan's hand with his teeth. Floyd screamed, of course, and everybody came running, but by the time they got that chimp to let up on Floyd's hand, he had bitten it up badly and broken a finger.

I had to anesthetize Floyd to dress his wounds and set his finger. Then I came every day to check on his hand and see how he was doing. I would talk to him real nice and pet him and console him, and he became very cooperative about letting me work on his hand. Even when it hurt him, he would yell and complain but rarely draw his hand away. He seemed to like the attention in spite of the pain. As soon as he saw me coming, he would hold the injured hand out to me.

Eventually Floyd's hand got well, of course. But the funny thing was that Floyd never forgot! Every time he saw me, he would run up to the bars of his cage and hold out his hand. I always went along with him. I'd take his hand, examine the finger and wiggle it a little bit, and talk to him—tell him what a good boy he was, and all. We kept up this routine for the rest of his life.

When I was a boy in Texas, we lived on a farm. I had three brothers, and none of them was the least bit interested in animals. I, on the other hand, loved them, so when we divided up the chores, I usually got to take care of our farm animals. I spent a lot of time with them alone. I think my love for our circus horses goes back to those days. I remember even then I fantasized about becoming a circus vet. Way back then, of course, the circus was still held in the big tent. Whenever it came through our part of Texas, my brothers and I always went, and it was something!

And so it was the most natural thing in the world for me to go to veterinary school at Texas A&M (Agricultural and Mechanical College). But of course, when I graduated, there were no jobs open for circus veterinarians—in fact, such a job just didn't exist. So I went into large-animal practice and did that for a number of years.

But I never gave up my determination to become a circus vet. Finally through some people I knew in Texas who had connections with Ringling Brothers, I heard the circus had decided to take on a full-time veterinarian, and I got the job. As far as I'm concerned, it's the most rewarding and colorful work in the world.

In all my years with the circus, I've only been injured once—that was my first year on the job. I carelessly walked too close to a panther cage. The panther reached out and took a swipe at me—caught me just on the joint of my chin. Nothing serious, just a very deep scratch. That taught me the lesson I've never once forgotten, and which has enabled me to do this job all these years: You've got to have respect for the animal. You have to remember that animals have their own integrity and their own ways. You have to know their ways. And though they may be more or less alike within their own species, each animal is still an individual. Whenever I address one of the circus animals, from the littlest dog to the biggest elephant, I have respect for that animal.

My favorite animals in the circus are the horses. Maybe it's because of my Texas childhood, but I love to treat them, take care of them, and watch them perform. They are so cooperative and beautiful to train. One thing about horses, though—and a lot of horse lovers are going to be mad at me for saying this—they are not too bright about some things. For example, horses seem to have very little common sense about their own welfare, about what will harm them. They injure themselves unnecessarily—stumble over obstacles that they could have easily avoided, for instance, or get themselves tangled up or stuck in dumb ways. But I still love the circus horses the best.

All our elephants are female; bull elephants would be hard to train and control. We get a lot of our elephants from the Portland Zoo, which breeds them. Most circus elephants are Indian, not African.

It is true that camels have rotten dispositions. Don't know why—they are just naturally a bit ornery. And they do spit—when they're angry, they can spit clear across the arena, almost. The saliva is very acid, and when it hits you on the skin, it can sting. And boy, if you should ever get hit in the eye, it could nearly blind you.

Naturally, the animals are much more confined when the circus is on the road than when they are in our winter quarters in Florida or in our large open acreage in Georgia. While the animals are in small cages, and subjected to crowds and noise, we have to take care to watch for signs of stress. Some animals are more claustrophobic than others, and we learn how to pick up their danger signals and do whatever we can to ease their stress.

One species that we breed pretty successfully in our Georgia location is giraffes. I've attended the birth of many giraffe calves—giraffes are members of the same family as cows, and the young are called calves. I'll never forget one particular obstetrical job I had with a giraffe. It was a breech birth. A breech is when the baby (doesn't matter if it's a calf, foal, or human baby) is in the wrong position in the birth canal and is trying to come out back first. In the case of four-legged animals, the normal birth position is head and forelegs first.

Without human help, both the mother animal and the infant often die in a breech-birth situation. The mother strains and strains trying to give birth, but can't get the baby past her pelvic bones. It's the same with human beings —a doctor or midwife has to reach in and turn the baby around into the correct headfirst position. With hooved animals, you might have the added danger of tearing the mother's uterus with the baby's hooves while you are turning it. But if the veterinarian or the farmer is careful, he can usually manage it.

Now, giraffes kick. So here I was confronted with a problem. The mother giraffe was standing up, and I had to perform this obstetrical function from behind, of course, which put me in a very vulnerable position. If she let fly with a hind leg while I was trying to help her, she could knock me senseless. Also, because of her height, I'd have to stand on something in order to reach her nether end, which was some two feet above my head.

So, here's what we did. I put the mother giraffe in a box stall with a wooden door that reached up almost to her behind, so if she kicked, she would kick the door. Then I got an elephant stool—one of those strong barrels that elephants stand on while they're performing—because it was sturdy and just the right height. And I got my helper to stand at her head and feed her crackers—a special kind of cracker which she loved. So he kept feeding her crackers and diverting her attention, and I stood on the elephant stool outside the door of the stall. I reached inside her and carefully turned the calf around, so it presented itself head and forelegs first. Once that was done, the baby giraffe sort of dived out quite easily while the mother was still chomping crackers. When she turned around and saw her baby in the straw at her feet, Nature took over—she forgot about the crackers and began to nuzzle and lick the calf. And I could get down off the elephant stool.

If you have heard, by the way, that giraffes have no voices, this is untrue. They don't have a big vocabulary of sounds, as many animals do, but they can make some. A mother giraffe will often make a sort of lowing sound to call her baby. These strange animals are fascinating to me —but then, I could say that about all the animals in the circus.

9. "I would hate never to see another tiger."

Elephants vary in personality like any other animals; there are among them intelligent ones and blithering idiots. As a whole, they have good memories, but they forget just like us.

—IVAN T. SANDERSON

The plight of the world's wild animals is a matter of interest and concern to a lot of people today, for many wild species are in serious danger of disappearing forever. One way some wild animals can be conserved is in zoos—that is, in good, professional, humane zoos.

Erik Kelner is the veterinarian of a large zoo; some 3,000 mammals, birds, and reptiles are under his care. He attends the zoo's animals as a highly trained farmer manages his flocks and herds, because that is what much of zoo medicine is all about. And of course he also gives individual medical care and treatment to any animal that needs it.

Dr. Kelner studied veterinary medicine for the technical skills and background he felt would be a valuable addition to his interest in and understanding of wildlife. He worked in zoos during his high school and college years, and also had some valuable experience on research teams studying wildlife in parts of South America and Africa. Because there are so few zoos that can support a full-time veterinarian, he had little hope of getting such a job when he finished veterinary school. But he was lucky.

Dr. Kelner has decided opinions about zoos—his own and others. This is what he has to tell us about the work of a zoo veterinarian.

In zoo medicine, one of the main disorders we have to be on the lookout for in our animals is trauma. Trauma, you know, means a serious hurt or damage—physical or mental, usually both. It can be caused by a physical injury, by a bad shock or fright, or by a sustained state of stress. Things that can traumatize a zoo animal are permanent overcrowding, boredom, lack of privacy, continual harassment (by people or by other animals). Boredom is a particularly severe stress factor for many captive animals. You see the big cats—lions, tigers, cheetahs, jaguars, and the like—pacing in their cages. They walk along the walls or in figure 8s; they may also chew on their own bodies or lick themselves raw. These are symptoms of boredom.

Stress presents a big problem when we have to examine and treat a sick zoo animal. If we use tranquilizers, as we usually do, we avoid stressing the animal but lose many of our diagnostic aids. Tranquilizers dull an animal's pain and diminish its alert responses. It's hard to pinpoint a tender area on a tranquilized animal, for example. Yet if we didn't use tranquilizers but restrained an animal with ropes or put it in a squeeze cage, we would stress it so much that we would have difficulty evaluating its pulse and breathing, even its body chemistry. So you can see how an animal that is continually or frequently under stress could eventually suffer trauma—damage to its heart, its stomach, its nervous system, whatever.

Sometimes trauma can be caused by a change of environment, or a change of diet. I'll give you a good example.

One time we got a new giant anteater, a young male named Reggie. We kept him in quarantine at the zoo's hospital for a few days, and then, since he was in good shape, we put him out in the exhibition area in a cage near the other anteaters. A few days later, I stopped by to see Reggie. Funny thing—he looked as though he'd lost weight. He was a real friendly guy who let you pet him, so I ran my hands over his back and sides, and sure enough, he felt thinner.

"How's Reggie eating?" I asked the keeper.

"Not good," the man said. "If he didn't get up an appetite by tomorrow, I was going to call you. I thought he just needed time to settle in."

"But he was eating okay when we had him in quarantine," I said.

"I'm about to feed the anteaters now—let's try him today and see if he'll eat," suggested the keeper. I followed him into the building where food for the anteaters was kept and prepared. I watched the keeper fixing the anteaters' food—a mixture of boiled eggs, ground meat, evaporated milk, Pablum, dog pellets, and water, with vitamins added. It suddenly hit me what could be wrong.

"Don't you put the food through the blender?" I asked.

"No. I've always fed it to them as is, just mixed. It doesn't look to me like it needs blending. The anteaters all like it just fine."

"We blended Reggie's at the hospital. Maybe at the zoo he came from, they also put the food through the blender," I said. "Try blending the food."

Reggie seemed hungry, and as soon as he tasted his food,

he ate it eagerly. The whole thing was the texture—while the unblended food looked and smelled just like the blended, the young anteater could tell the difference and would have none of it.

If Reggie had gone on not eating, in a few more days he would have died. The immediate cause of death would probably have been pneumonia or some other infection, but the real cause would have been starvation—brought on by being traumatized by that slight change in his diet.

Most of the time, however, my work is not the treatment of individual animals, but a matter of management. That is one big difference between us zoo veterinarians and those in private practice. When several animals in a herd show symptoms, I look for changes in their environment. Any treatment I give is to the whole herd.

Just last year, we had a bad situation with our elk. The entire herd, which had been a good healthy bunch, began to show signs of malnutrition—in spite of their regular, balanced diet. I checked their site and couldn't find anything wrong at first. Then one day I noticed them drinking at a pond at the far end of their grounds instead of at their water trough, and I got an idea. I discovered their watering trough had a clogged drain which the keeper hadn't reported. The water in the trough became stagnant, and so the elk had taken to drinking out of the pond instead. The pond was loaded with parasites, and the elk had become malnourished because of the parasites. We had to fence off the pond, fix the drain of the trough, of course, and treat the whole herd for the parasites, or we would have lost every one of them.

I make rounds daily and get to every exhibit in the zoo at least once a week. But I have to rely tremendously on the keepers. Some keepers are great—they really know their animals, really care about them, and are aware and perceptive. You can depend on them completely. But of course, some keepers are unreliable, don't show up for work, don't really pay attention to their animals. Unfortunately, the veterinarian does not hire or train the keepers; we all work for the zoo.

The minute you put a wild animal into captivity, you subject it to varying degrees of stress. That is why I much prefer to see zoos acquire animals from other zoos, or breed their own, rather than buy animals that have been captured in the wild and subjected to the treatment they suffer at the hands of animal importers.

Yet zoos have a problem in that a great many species will not reproduce in cages. The answer may be breeding farms —large acreages where animals live in conditions that approximate their natural habitats. But these are few and expensive, and—in the case of primates—the animals can't breed fast enough to keep up with the needs of the research centers.

The Endangered Species Act of 1973 restricts the importation of some animals that are facing imminent extinction. Zoos are increasingly going to have to rely on themselves to perpetuate many of the world's exotic animals.

Humanitarians tend to regard zoos as no better than prisons for animals. But if you think about it, the life of most animals in their natural environment is no bed of roses. It's a continual struggle to stay alive—to find water, shelter, to find food without being killed as food for somebody else.

Imagine the stress an antelope lives in all its life! It is subject to predation from so many other animals that it can't even venture to a water hole without being on a life-or-death alert. And when a wild animal is sick or injured, forget it. Even in those big game refuges or wildlife preservation farms, a sick animal usually won't get noticed until it's near death.

Today, wild animals are being continually destroyed, partly through hunting and trapping, but largely through the steady decrease in wilderness land where they can support themselves. The encroachments of human habitation and industrial pollution are finishing off the wildlife of the whole world. One single timber wolf needs twenty square miles full of the same game he has to kill to keep himself alive. Bengal tigers—those few that are left—each need 300 square miles. So it is easy to imagine the not-so-distant end of wildlife that naturalists are predicting. Good zoos offer the only alternative to extinction for most of our present wild species. I would hate never to see another tiger.

I believe zoos should have the same stature and professionalism as botanical gardens or natural history museums. They should be educational and research institutions first, and recreation places second. An art museum does not have a carnival atmosphere; neither should a zoo.

A good zoo tries to approximate the natural habitat of its animals as closely as possible. Freedom with control; spacious, naturalistic environments instead of sterile, concrete cages. One type of cage that should be replaced is the round cage where the animal can get no privacy, no place to hide from people staring at it. Some knowledge of wildlife is helpful, even essential, to zoo veterinarians. You have to know, for instance, that lemurs will do well only in cages tall enough to permit high perches, because they are arboreal, or tree-living, creatures and like the feeling of space under them. Or that some species of deer do better with a gravel floor under them than a dirt floor. Zoos today are cooperating with each other to learn how best to preserve and perpetuate animals in captivity.

In the past, for example, zookeepers would sometimes

put one male animal in a cage with a female of the same species, and when they failed to mate, would wonder why. Now we know that for many species to reproduce you have to let the males and females live together in groups, as they do in the wild. We really know so little about wild animals in their natural state, that we're only beginning to know what's *normal* for any given species.

When I first came to work for the zoo, I didn't even know the precise physiology of some of our species. The second day I was in my job, I was called to look at a brown pelican. I went out to the pelican cage and found the keeper holding the sick bird. Well, I had never examined a pelican before.

"He's not eating well," said the keeper. "He seems listless."

Of course, I was trying to make a good impression, so I took a complete history and started to check over the pelican very carefully. When I palpated him—felt his chest and stomach—I discovered what I thought to be serious trouble.

"He has a bad subcutaneous emphysema in his chest," I announced. "That means air underneath the skin." I went through the whole description of subcutaneous emphysema, and what it could mean. I was truly concerned.

The keeper listened very attentively and politely. When I got all through, he shook his head and said, "Well, you know, Doc, I always thought it was his air pocket. I've been working here for twenty-two years, and every pelican I've ever seen has an air pocket in its chest. They're all built that way—they need that air pocket for diving. It cushions the shock when they hit the water."

Of course. A pelican flies rather high over the water, then, when he spots a fish, dives kerplunk with a great splash.

For me, this was what you call on-the-job learning, I guess. I've forgotten now what we did for that pelican, but I know he recovered faster than I did!

People are sometimes awed by the fact that a zoo veterinarian has to treat so many different animals. They range in weight from five grams to 8,000 pounds. A newborn polar bear weighs less than two pounds; a baby rhino can weigh two hundred. But in giving them medical care, I am much less concerned with their differences than with their similarities. In spite of some unique species variations, they all have hearts, lungs, stomachs, organ systems, endocrine systems. Exotic animals are not physiologically different from farm animals or pet animals.

Every so often a veterinarian in small-animal practice will phone me up to ask my advice on how to treat somebody's unusual pet.

"I've never had an ocelot (or a skunk, perhaps, or a kinkajou) for a patient before," he'll say. "It seems to have a respiratory infection. How much antibiotic should I administer?"

He always seems surprised when I say, "Treat it as you would an ordinary dog or cat of that size—it's the same class of mammal."

It's especially hard for the general public to imagine zoo veterinary work, because so much of it is unexciting maintenance and research. Take a typical day's work—yesterday is a good example.

In the morning I anesthetized an elderly margay and did some necessary dental work. Then I paid a call to the reptile house to see a sick turtle—the keeper reported that he seemed sluggish and disoriented and was swimming in a corkscrew pattern. I discovered he had fluid in his body cavity, so I drew some out to send to the lab for analysis, gave him a shot of antibiotics, and had him moved to shallow water so he wouldn't drown. I also checked an iguana who was recovering from superficial burns he had suffered from sitting too near a heat lamp. Then I drove over to the pony barn and gave our eleven ponies shots of antibiotics—they had a respiratory virus, and we wanted to head off anything worse that might develop.

But the most satisfying work I did all day, really, was preparing a statistical analysis of the breeding problems of one of our groups of penguins. This doesn't sound exciting, but it is very valuable research. In zoo medicine, you study the behavior of animals and observe such factors as play, aggression, and sex, and you get to know how these habits are related to their health. You also learn how diet, population density, privacy—or lack of it—can affect the health of the animals.

I recently read about an innovation that progressive zoos may make in the future. At a zoo in the Midwest, there is an experiment going which is aimed at restoring the keen hunting instinct of wild animals. Zoo animals are of course fed at regular times every day. When a wild animal gets used to having its dinner handed to it, it becomes complacent and lazy, and its hunting instinct is blunted from lack of use. Temperamentally, it is no longer the same animal.

Well, at this zoo I read about, the cages where two pumas are kept have been rigged up with mechanical marmots that scurry from one hole to another. To activate the marmots, each puma has to jump onto a "stalking limb" over a marmot hole and wait. When the mechanical marmot makes a run for it, the puma pounces. If he's fast enough, a device delivers meat to him. If he's too slow, no dinner. He has to stalk again. The zoo plans to set up similar experiments with other animals that live by hunting, to keep life more normal for them.

It's ironic that we should be contriving methods to keep wildness in our zoo animals. But I think anything a zoo can do to approximate the natural life of its animals will be good for the animals and at the same time keep them more authentic members of their various species. The public will get a better idea of the true wonder of our wildlife.

Another zoo—the Portland, Oregon, zoo—has instituted some elaborate setups which teach animals to pull levers and push buttons to get food, as part of the zoo's ongoing study of animal intelligence and behavior. These systems give the animals something to do and relieve their boredom, as well as stimulate interest on the part of the public. I think there is a lot of new thinking going on in zoo management and in zoo medicine that should bring about great changes for the better.

10.

"So little is known about sea mammals, every procedure is a first."

When dolphins lead the ships by day in the oldest
sea
No tremor of change trembles their light where they
lie
Clear and in long trajectory follow the arc of the
world. . . .
They rise on the wake of the eastward vessel out of
Gibraltar,
They stand over water, slim, with their flippers of
balance spread like arms or wings. . . .
—BREWSTER GHISELIN

There's a very small, very new specialty in veterinary medicine: the study and medical care of sea mammals—the whales, dolphins, seals, and other warm-blooded, air-breathing animals that live in aquariums or aquatic zoos but breathe air. This work is becoming increasingly important. If human beings continue to pollute the waters of the world, then the warnings of some scientists will come true very fast, and there will no longer be any natural marine life—animal, plant, or other. Captive creatures will be the only ones to survive, and all the knowledge we have about them will be essential in conserving and perpetuating them. The few veterinarians who have taken up marine mammal medicine are truly pioneers today.

One of them is Alex Tombeck, who divides his time between his small-animal practice in a suburb of New York and his consulting work with marine mammals that are exhibited in zoos and aquariums. Instead of wearing a white coat, a suit, or even work clothes, Dr. Tombeck is likely to practice his specialty in a wetsuit —the tight-fitting rubber suit that divers wear. He speaks of his work with enthusiasm.

Once when I was on a skin-diving vacation in the Florida Keys, I got a call from someone I knew at a local ocean-arium asking me to examine a sick dolphin. When I got out there, I discovered that the dolphin's trainer, a young woman named Sarah, was almost sick herself with worry.

"He's listless and off his feed," she said. "I don't know what's wrong with him or what to do for him. He's just not himself. Please try to help him!" People who work with whales and dolphins have a really close relationship with their animals, as close as any love between people and dogs.

The first thing I had to do, of course, was examine the animal, who was in a big deep-water pen. We had to get him into the shallow water in one corner, and since it was after hours, there was nobody around to help us corral him. So Sarah and I took a large net between us and slowly dragged it across the pen. It took us two hours to get the dolphin, who was called Duffy, into the corner, where Sarah could grab him and hang on to him.

The animal showed signs of thiamin deficiency—a condition not unusual among captive marine mammals who are fed a diet of only one kind of fish. I gave it an injection of thiamin, which is a B-complex vitamin.

The next day I went back to give Duffy another injection. I thought, "Oh Lord, it will take another two hours to catch him, I'll have to do this every day for a week, and here I am on vacation." But I was resigned to it; I did want to get that dolphin well.

Sarah was waiting by Duffy's pen.

"Could we get some help in herding him into the corner today, so it won't take us so long?" I asked.

"Yes, we can. But let me try something else first," said Sarah. She called Duffy. The animal swam past her slowly, looked up at us, and circled a bit sluggishly. Sarah pointed to the shallow corner. Would you believe that dolphin swam immediately into the corner? I waded up to him, and he submitted quietly to the injection I gave him. Then he swam away.

This went on every day. All I had to do was appear, and Sarah would call to Duffy, who would swim into the shallow corner and wait for me. As the week went on, Duffy obviously began to feel much better.

"He's back to his regular eating habits and seems to be fine," reported Sarah happily.

Well, on the last day, I guess Duffy thought things had gone far enough. He swam into the corner as soon as Sarah called him, and waited for me as usual. I gave him the shot, but as I was drawing the needle out of him that last time, he turned around and nipped me. He knocked me off my feet in the waist-deep water, leaving me splashing and struggling, still holding the syringe. Meanwhile, Duffy swam gaily off, a healthy dolphin with a crude sense of humor—and no feeling of gratitude whatsoever.

I grew up on Long Island and as a child had the usual pets—dogs, cats, tropical fish. I always wanted to be a veterinarian. I think I was strongly influenced by the Dr. Doolittle books—I thought how great it would be to be able to talk to animals. Becoming a veterinarian was the closest thing to it I could think of.

I worked on a farm during the summers I was in high school and then went to "ag" school at Cornell. After two years I was accepted into the veterinary college, and graduated in 1957. I spent my two years in the Air Force working with sentry dogs. Today I put in five days a week at my small-animal practice, see about twenty animals a day. But my first love is my work with aquatic mammals.

I've always loved the sea—I'm a fisherman and skin diver. And in fact, there was a time in my life when I thought of going back to school and getting a Ph.D. in Marine Biology. But rather than put in another five years in college, I started to study and treat marine mammals out at the aquarium, using my experience as a veterinarian in a way that satisfies my interest in aquatic life. For the last six years, I've been learning on the job there, and now I have as much experience as most people in the marine mammal field.

You can't earn a living just in aquatic mammal medicine —there simply aren't enough specimens in captivity to support the specialty. I don't make money in it. It's full of problems—but what a challenge! There are only a few veterinarians involved in this work—maybe fifty in the whole world. We have an organization called the International Association for Aquatic Mammal Medicine, and I attended its annual conference recently. There were people there from the Netherlands, England, the Soviet Union, Canada, New Zealand—all over. Everybody's knowledge and experience are important and contribute to the small sum of information we have. Almost every time one of us works on these animals, it's a first.

Marine mammals are like other mammals in some ways, and very different in others. They once lived on land, you know. All life originated in the sea, millions of years ago, and in the process of evolution, many creatures moved up onto land. At some point later, marine mammals reversed the evolutionary direction, returned to the sea, and adapted themselves to the water—although they do of course breathe air.

The two main classifications of sea mammals are the pinipeds—fin-footed animals such as seals and walruses—and the cetaceans, which include dolphins and the many species of whales. Dolphins are sometimes called "porpoises," although technically the porpoise is a different sea animal; the creatures you see in aquariums are dolphins.

Dolphins have always had an unusual, friendly relationship with humans. There are stories going back hundreds of years about dolphins saving the lives of shipwrecked sailors. Surviving sailors often used to report that they were pushed ashore by a large sea creature. Some tales about dolphins are probably folklore, but others are undoubtedly true. I think it was the great Roman naturalist Pliny the Elder who wrote in the first century A.D. that the dolphin is the only animal friendly to man who has no need of him whatsoever. Some people who work with dolphins report instances of what they think is ESP between themselves and their particular animals.

Dolphins are playful—with each other and with people. There are documented cases of friendly ones hanging around beaches where people swim. I read several accounts of a dolphin who used to appear off a certain beach in New Zealand, swim with the people, and let the children ride on him and tow him. He would show up for a couple of months every year and hang around. Then he'd disappear and not be seen again until the following year. It was a marvelous instance of a wild animal coming to be with human beings of its own accord. Nobody ever tried to tame him; he just acted on his own feelings of affinity and friendliness toward people.

This dolphin was greatly loved and famous all over New

Zealand. When he died—they found his body on a beach, finally—the local people had a funeral for him.

Sometimes when you're out in a boat in waters where there are dolphins, one will suddenly appear and ride your bow waves and swim close to the boat in a friendly way. I can't think of any other wild animal that will do that— hang around people out of choice.

Dolphins are highly intelligent. The weight of their brain in ratio to the weight of their body is not much less than that of human beings. There are other factors in intelligence, of course, but brain weight in ratio to body weight is one important factor. A dolphin's brain is also comparable to a person's in complexity.

This combination of intelligence and affinity for man makes dolphins highly trainable. The Navy is doing experimental work with them to make use of some of their special abilities. For example, dolphins have more than one highly specialized sonar system. Sonar, you know, means bouncing a sound off an object in order to measure its distance. Dolphins have fantastic echo-locating ability— we're just beginning to know how remarkable it is. Also, these animals can dive rapidly to tremendous depths—as much as 200 feet—and come up in seconds, with no adverse physiological effects. They don't get the "bends" that human beings are subject to when they come up from deep water skin diving. We don't know why. The Navy trains dolphins to retrieve on command; they'll bring up sunken bombs, objects from sunken submarines, whatever. Unfortunately, a cutback in appropriations has narrowed this remarkable work. I think there's a tremendous need for research on the sea—not just by veterinarians, but by people from all scientific fields—to discover what the sea can offer for humankind.

A couple of years ago some Eskimos up in the Canadian Arctic were out fishing when they noticed an animal about five feet long sort of nestling up against their boat. They discovered it was a baby narwhale. Those are the whales with a single, long ivory tusk—at least the adult males have the tusk. The narwhale is believed to be the animal that the legendary unicorn is based on. Anyway, the mother narwhale had apparently been killed, and the baby saw the long shadow of the boat and came up to see if it was its mother. The Eskimos had no trouble capturing the little whale and bringing it to shore.

The local Canadian game warden came along and decided to try to save the poor creature. But when he started to feed it some sardines, the baby tried to suck on his hand, and he realized it was too young to eat; it was still nursing. He called the famous Coney Island aquarium to find out what to do.

Another veterinarian and I decided to fly up to Canada in a small plane and bring the baby narwhale back. We packed it in wet cloths and brought it down to New York in the plane with us. Then we were faced with the problem of formula—who knew what the formula for narwhale milk was?

We did the best we could, and the baby narwhale drank what we gave it, but in a few days it died. I think the setback it suffered between the death of its mother and the time we finally fed it had weakened the narwhale beyond help.

Recently some people found a beached harbor seal and brought it to the aquarium. Whenever a sea animal is beached and sick enough to be captured, it is usually too sick to save. The harbor seal died of pneumonia—which we believe is a common disease of its species. For one thing, seal rookeries are very dirty places—I suspect a lot

of seals become ill from the filth in their own rookeries.
Thousands of seals will congregate in the same place, which
becomes overcrowded, overpopulated. They urinate and
defecate everywhere of course, and then the pups are born
and roll in the mess. I think rookeries must be breeding
grounds for disease, especially bacterial and verminous
pneumonia.

There is a strict law now to protect marine mammals—
you can't even take a dead one that's washed up on the
beach without a permit. This law will put a lot of people
who were hunting them out of business. Good, I say. It
might be defensible to take a limited number of marine
mammals for display in excellent zoos where ideal conditions exist—but even that's a risk, because they suffer from
stress and boredom in captivity, the same as other caged
wild animals. Marine mammals need a lot of water room,
and if there are too many of them in too small a pool, they
suffer.

Aquatic mammals in zoos are prey to many of the same
diseases other mammals get—respiratory infections, viral
infections, bacterial infections, worms, fleas (a special kind
of water flea). They also suffer from swallowing rubber
balls and other foreign objects that some people are foolish
enough to throw into their cages.

Even strict conservation laws can't save many of our
marine species now. The biggest whales are the most endangered. It's already too late for the killer whales and
pilot whales, and probably for the blue whales also. Whales
are the largest animals that have ever lived on earth, and
go back to prehistoric times. Compared to them the dino-
saurs were small. Blue whales grow to be 100, even 120,
feet long, too big to keep in captivity. The blue whales are
so endangered today that many biologists think they will
never reproduce fast enough to survive as a species. I think

it's a shame that this unique animal will become extinct in our time.

In some places—mainly Eskimo lands and parts of northern Japan—whales are an important part of the people's diet, and may even be their means of survival. That's why some Eskimo villages are permitted under the international treaties to take a limited number of whales each year. The Japanese have so far refused to sign the international agreements limiting whaling. They claim that telling the northern Japanese to stop eating whale meat would be like telling Americans to stop eating beef.

Harpooned whales die a very slow, bloody, painful death. I personally would like to see all whaling stopped. Period. But you have to consider the needs of people who depend on this animal, and I don't know of a solution. Conservationists point out that there are cheap substitutes available for all products made from whales. It would certainly be worthwhile to develop them.

Because of my work with sea mammals, I become involved in ecological, philosophical, economic, and political issues that most vets are not affected by. I don't mind—I'll do whatever I can to save these wonderful creatures.

11.

"We might find the cause and cure for cancer."

Physiological experiment on animals is justifiable for real investigation, but not for mere damnable and detestable curiosity.

—CHARLES DARWIN

Medical research attracts a number of veterinarians who work with teams of physicians and other scientists on solving the mysteries of disease. The similarities between animals and humans in physiology and in the diseases they contract make this alliance of professions a productive one. Veterinarians conduct and participate in research at hospitals, medical centers, universities, and drug companies.

Geoffrey Heller is the chief of a team of three veterinarians who work together in the veterinary cancer unit of a large medical center. Medical research is slow, painstaking work; the rewards are elusive, and the victories are infrequent. Here Dr. Heller tries to make what he does understandable to the nonscientist.

It was hard for me to make the decision to go into research work full time. I really like animals, and sometimes

I miss working with them. My two partners, Rosemary and John, work here at the laboratory part time and spend several days a week at two small-animal hospitals, in special cancer clinics where animals with cancer are treated. Their clinical work is the applied end of our research; they take our laboratory discoveries, try them on animals with cancer, and keep track of the results.

Here at the lab, we have no animals; all our work is done with microscopes and other research instruments and machines. It is rarely dramatic or exciting. Yet, we think what we are doing will possibly bring a real breakthrough in the control and conquest of cancer. It's enormously thrilling when you think about it in the large sense rather than as a day-by-day routine.

How did I get into this kind of research? Well, my favorite subject in veterinary school at the University of Pennsylvania was immunology—that probably awakened my interest in research. Immunology, you know, is the study and science that deals with the body's inborn protections against disease. I worked for two summers in the laboratory at school on a research grant—on my own projects, but under the direction of my professor. It was so gratifying that I realized research was what I liked most of all.

When I graduated, I put in a fifteen-month clinical internship at an ASPCA hospital. I wasn't completely sold on staying in the laboratory the rest of my life. I wanted to learn about the clinical and applied aspect of veterinary medicine before I started to look for a job in research.

Then I heard about the work being done here toward finding the way to make organisms immune to cancer. I heard they were putting together a veterinary medical team to be headed by a doctor I'd always admired. I applied for a staff position, and they hired me.

My colleague John Sapinsky was hired because he had been doing special work in oncology during his residency at an animal hospital after graduation from the University of Illinois Veterinary School. Oncology is the study of tumors. You see a lot of tumors on dogs and cats, and the malignant, or cancerous, ones are much like human cancers. I suspect John came to work here for the same reason I did—the challenge of searching out the cause of cancer and its cure.

Rosemary Quinn was snapped up right out of veterinary school. When the big guns here at the cancer center were putting together our particular research unit, they searched the veterinary schools for the most promising person to complete the team with John and me. Rosemary was picked out of hundreds of graduates all over the country. She had a spectacular academic record at Cornell and had done some research in endocrinology—the study of glands and secretions—while she was still in school. She had had several job offers, but decided to team up with John and me. We three have great respect for each other.

Some people are surprised to learn that veterinarians are engaged in medical research in human diseases. But historically, human medicine and veterinary medicine have often been linked—in fact, in earliest times they were virtually interchangeable. Physicians often treated animals, and it was not unusual for a veterinarian to be called to attend a sick or injured person. The two professions became separate after the eighteenth century in terms of practice, but cooperative research has continued—especially in microbiology and immunology.

Diphtheria vaccine and tetanus vaccine were developed by a veterinarian. The work of vets in chemotherapy laid the groundwork for the conquests of leprosy, yellow fever, malaria, cholera, and certain types of tuberculosis.

Today some three hundred vets work in biomedical research for the Department of Health, Education, and Welfare alone. Veterinarians have pioneered in orthopedics and anesthesia, in ophthalmology, in nearly every medical specialty. So there is really nothing unusual, after all, about the fact that John, Rosemary, and I do research at a human medical center.

People often ask me about my work, and when I tell them what I do, they seem shocked.

"How can you bear to take a dog or cat and inject it with cancer cells, or whatever you do to cause it to develop cancer?" they'll ask.

I explain that we never do that. We don't have to cause a healthy animal to develop cancer. We only use animals that already have cancer, animals at the clinics where my two partners work. Cancer is so common among dogs and cats that you see a lot of it in any place with a large population of pets. All the animals we work with are referred to the cancer clinics for therapy by private veterinarians or are brought there directly by their owners. We treat nearly 2,000 animals a year.

In the old days, all you could do for an animal that had any form of cancer was to operate on it—try to cut the malignancy out—or put the animal to sleep. Now, we try surgery, radiation, or drugs—those are the traditional forms of cancer treatment—and sometimes we have been successful in combining them in new ways. But more important, we also try some new forms of therapy.

Right now I'm working on immunotherapy at the lab. Immunotherapy is the attempt to stimulate the body's own defense mechanisms to destroy malignant cells. We also are experimenting with serum therapy—using the fluid portion of blood in a way we have discovered sometimes kills cancer cells.

One important part of our work involves a type of cancer called feline leukemia. We have discovered that feline leukemia, like some other cat diseases, is caused by a virus. It's a whole new concept—the idea of a type of cancer being infectious. If we can develop a vaccine against it, we will really be making significant progress.

Although feline leukemia is much like human leukemia, there is no evidence that a person can get leukemia from a cat that has feline leukemia. But, it is known to be contagious from cat to cat.

Our work doesn't go on in a vacuum. All information—everything we learn, every success or failure we have—is coordinated with other research and made available to physicians treating human cancer patients. Other groups similar to our unit, groups at hospitals and veterinary schools, are collaborating with us. The immunological approach to cancer is new and very promising—we are really excited about it.

Like many other people in research, we do have a continual worry about grants. There's always the possibility that the funds from the organizations that support our research will run out, and we won't get a new grant to continue our work. If that happens, I can speak for the three of us: not only will we be out of our jobs, our hearts will be broken. It will make us feel that all our work against this terrible disease has been useless.

12. "We brought the epidemic under control."

Animals are not brethren, they are not underlings; they are other nations, caught with ourselves in the net of life and time.

—HENRY BESTON

About 2,400 veterinarians in the United States work for the Department of Agriculture. They comprise only about 6 percent of the total number of veterinarians —yet what they do affects every person living in this country, and hundreds of millions of animals. These doctors are in what is called "regulatory" veterinary medicine; they administer laws and perform services that affect the health and well-being of virtually all animals raised for meat, all poultry, animals imported to this country, animals sold and exhibited, animals used in research. Without these veterinarians, you could not eat a hamburger or drink a glass of milk without the risk of getting sick, maybe dying. Although the veterinarians in regulatory veterinary medicine have tremendous responsibilities that protect the health of everybody in the country, most of us know very little about their work.

Charles Smedley and Jane Talbot are veterinarians in the Animal and Plant Health Inspection Service, a branch of the U.S. Department of Agriculture. They work in an office building not far from Washington, D. C. Dr. Smedley holds a senior position in the Emergency Programs division, while Dr. Talbot heads a division that proposes and enforces laws for the humane treatment of animals.

Dr. Smedley speaks first:

When we hear of an outbreak of a communicable animal disease, we sometimes have to work like detectives and sometimes like an army engaged in battle. First we must quickly find the source—that's where the detective work comes in—and then we have to muster all our personnel and equipment to combat it. The disease becomes an enemy that can move fast and kill. Two years ago we had a serious emergency that was a good example of this.

The first news we had that something was wrong was a call from the State Diagnostic Laboratory in southern California.

"We think there's trouble ahead," one of the technicians said. "A farmer came in here yesterday with several chickens from what was left of his backyard flock. He had lost 95 percent of his chickens in one week, and was really hurting. He thought they might have been poisoned, but he couldn't figure out with what. We've been running tests on the chickens he brought us, and it doesn't look good."

"What do you think they've got?" I asked.

"Looks like exotic Newcastle disease," the fellow in California said. "We've already notified all the agriculture agents in the area to be on the alert, but we thought we ought to warn you people there in Washington. You'll probably want to get ready for some action."

You'd better believe it! Exotic Newcastle is a deadly virus disease that is not native to this country but can be brought in by birds imported from foreign countries. If it gets started, it spreads like wildfire, wiping out every bird over a wide area. We alerted our agents in the Southwest.

Next day, a scientist from the Diagnostic Laboratory called back. "Yep, that's it," he said. "Big trouble."

We went into action immediately, notifying all our agents to track down every case of sick chickens and try to stop the spread of the disease. In just that one small area of southern California, there are over 40 million birds on big chicken farms and in small backyard flocks—an ideal situation for a disease like Newcastle to spread rapidly. We also told our investigators to try to discover how this disease had started. That first farmer's chickens must have caught it from a foreign source, but how?

Within a matter of months, the death rate among southern California chickens was extremely high. At that point, the Secretary of Agriculture declared the situation a national emergency. Things were bad in southern California, but if exotic Newcastle started to spread across the country, it could kill practically every chicken in the United States and wipe out the poultry industry.

Once the state of national emergency was declared, we were given the authority—and the funds—to take strong measures. We mobilized over 3,290 personnel in the fight.

Animal Health Inspection Service agents started vaccination programs and were vaccinating chickens like crazy —we used up over 112 million doses of vaccine. It is not a totally effective vaccine, but it was the best weapon we had. And whenever we discovered a chicken who already had the disease, it would be slaughtered. We killed almost 12 million birds!

In the meantime, one of the epidemiologists tracking down the source came across it, right in the neighborhood of the small farm where the disease had first been noted. During his investigations, he discovered an importer of exotic pet birds a few hundred yards away. This importer brought in macaws, parrots, and parakeets from several foreign countries. Yes, an entire shipment of his birds had died recently. That was it, of course. Though the pet birds had had no direct contact with the flock of chickens nearby, it was close enough for exotic Newcastle to spread to them.

I'm glad to tell you we were able to bring that exotic Newcastle epidemic under control; it never spread out of California. There have been a few small outbreaks since then in other parts of the country—Texas, Florida, New York (we recently had to close down a pet shop in New York when we discovered a case)—but those cases were brought in independently, they weren't related to the big California epidemic.

When the Department of Agriculture has to kill chickens or livestock to control an epidemic, we compensate the farmers for their loss, pay them what their animals are worth. That Newcastle epidemic in California cost 56 million dollars to eradicate. But when you consider that if the epidemic had gone unchecked it would have cost the country—and that means ultimately the consumer—over 230 million dollars each year that the epidemic lasted, I'd say the price was worth it, wouldn't you?

When I was a boy in Texas, I got a job helping a cowboy who, though untrained, was pretty good at most things having to do with livestock. He treated their illnesses and even performed simple operations. It seemed to me like a fine way to earn a living, so I went to veterinary school at Texas A & M University—the vet school was and still is part of the Agriculture College.

At that time the Mexican government and the USDA Bureau of Animal Industry were trying to eradicate foot-and-mouth disease, a fatal disease of cattle. Thousands of cattle were brought into the United States from Mexico every year, and even with cattle inspection at every point along the border, there was still a chance that the disease could slip into this country. If that happened, our entire livestock industry would be threatened. It was more efficient and less expensive for the U.S. Government to join with Mexico in fighting the disease *there*.

So I joined the Bureau of Animal Industry and spent five years in Mexico. I learned the language, got to know the people, and enjoyed living there very much. We were finally successful in eradicating foot-and-mouth disease.

The Bureau of Animal Industry, forerunner of the Animal and Plant Health Inspection Service, was started by Congress after a bad cattle disease rampaged here in the late 1800s. A British ship had brought in a cow with pleuropneumonia, which quickly spread among our cattle that were awaiting shipment overseas. This was before shipboard refrigeration was developed to the point where frozen meat could be shipped, so beef was sent to our overseas markets on the hoof. When the British, French, and German port inspectors discovered our cattle had pleuropneumonia, they wouldn't let the animals into their countries, and we lost our export markets. The Bureau of Animal Industry was set up to protect the health of our domestic animals.

You should see what a thorough operation we run today in Emergency Programs. We know every important detail of what's happening in animal health all over the country —what disease has broken out and where; whether it has spread to another state or county; how many animals are affected; how many farmers are involved; what kind of money and how many people are needed to stop it. We have an extensive information-retrieval library; all the published material on animal diseases that call for emergency measures is on microfilm. Any information we need is available to us by computer in a matter of seconds, and our transmitting machines can send the information to our veterinarians in the field in minutes.

I think our work here in Emergency Programs is very sophisticated and efficient; I get enormous satisfaction from being part of it.

Now Jane Talbot speaks:

When I was a young girl, I was a real horse lover—and still am. I had my own horse, used to ride in shows, and in fact went to veterinary school because I wanted to be a horse veterinarian. I was among the first women to graduate from a veterinary college.

I started out doing a stint as a meat-inspection veterinarian. Back then, we—myself and other inspectors all over the country—discovered almost a million pounds a day of unsafe meat that would have been sold to the public if we hadn't prevented it.

The reason I became a meat-inspection veterinarian was to increase my knowledge of the pathology of large-animal diseases. There's no better place to learn pathology than on the slaughterhouse floor. But in those days we didn't have the humane laws we have now, and I'm telling you, the screams of the shackled animals hung up by their legs waiting to be killed was more than I could bear. Their suffering was terrible. Meat inspection is very important work, but I don't know any vet who enjoys the killing related to it, even today when it is less brutal. I had to inspect the animals before and after they were killed. The lambs and calves were so innocent; they'd nuzzle me and try to suck my finger as I examined them. The next time I'd see them, they'd be dead.

Nowadays, at least, animals are stunned before they are shackled up to bleed out. In addition to examining the animals for health, our Department of Agriculture veterinarians are responsible for seeing that the humane laws are respected. One meat company, Hormel, kills their hogs in an especially humane way. They move them one by one through a tunnel in which carbon dioxide is released. This puts the animals peacefully to sleep, and when they are killed they never feel a thing. Some other packers use the carbon dioxide tunnel for sheep and calves. I personally wish they could use it for cattle too.

Department of Agriculture veterinarians also test milk cows for tuberculosis. Some types of TB that cattle get are transferable to people. Back in the twenties and thirties, this was a real danger. There were cases in which a meat inspection veterinarian spotted TB in a cow and alerted the Public Health Service. When the people on the farm the cow came from were checked, it was found that they too had TB, which can be communicated either from drinking the milk or eating the meat of infected cows. That was one of the reasons the Bureau of Animal Industry—our ancestor organization—came into being. TB is rare in dairy cattle today because most milk comes from large dairy farms on which the cows have been TB tested and the sanitary and health laws are enforced.

I learned a lot as a meat-inspection veterinarian but was glad to go into private practice after a few years. I went into large-animal practice and loved it. But unfortunately, about seven years later, I had a bad accident. I didn't get kicked—that's the common danger of vets in large-animal practice—I was run over by a bull. I was in a cattle pen vaccinating cows when somebody accidentally let a bull into the pen. I was trampled. When I got out of the hospital, I decided to go back into regulatory medicine. But this time I went into humane work because it was more appealing to me.

One of the laws our division is entrusted with enforcing is the Horse Protection Act of 1970, which is intended to outlaw the soring of the Tennessee Walking Horse. Soring is a very cruel practice of injuring the feet of these famous show horses so they pick their feet up smartly in the show ring. The owners and trainers use chemicals, chains, or special painful boots on the part of the horses' front feet called the pastern—the area between the hoof line and the first joint. When a horse's front feet are sore, he will reach with his hind feet to take his weight off the painful front feet, and this gives the appearance of gliding, which goes over big with the judges. There's a lot of money involved in the competition of these valuable horses. The Horse Protection Act makes it illegal to "use any method or device on a horse's feet for the purpose of altering his gait that will cause him pain or discomfort when he is moving."

Unfortunately, the act has many loopholes, and strengthening it has become difficult because of political pressures from opposition groups. Even so, our inspectors do the best they can. We have made over 350 cases. So far we have won twelve criminal cases and fifty civil ones. The criminal penalty is a fine of up to $2,000 and a year in jail, or both; the civil penalty is up to $1,000.

One thing that has helped is our new detection machine. Sometimes you can't see with the naked eye that a horse's feet have been sored—the owners have become so clever at disguising it that even when you can tell by a horse's unnatural gait that his feet hurt him badly, you can't find a mark on him. But our new infrared heat-sensing camera can. Injured tissue sends off heat. When we suspect a horse has been sored, we photograph his feet with this camera. The owners know that when we catch them, they're in trouble, so it has some deterrent effect.

Another responsibility of the Animal Care staff is administering the Animal Welfare Act, which prohibits cruelty to animals among wholesale breeders, dealers, and exhibitors—from tiny roadside circuses on up to large zoos. The inspectors have no control over retail pet shops that sell to the public except those that sell exotic animals such as monkeys, ferrets, and ocelots. But we can actually close down a wholesale dealer who doesn't provide humane care and decent conditions for the animals he has for sale.

Animal Care inspectors also supervise the shipment of animals. Last year they passed out over 100 violations at airports alone. And they inspect research laboratories to see that the laboratory animals have adequate veterinary care and are not caused unnecessary pain or experimented on without appropriate painkillers. Every year, research laboratories have to file a report telling the number of animals they have used and for what purpose.

Our humane laws are far from perfect, and the Animal Care department has only a limited number of inspectors. But they do a pretty good job as far as they can within our laws, and there's no question that they do prevent considerable suffering.

The first veterinarians in the Department of Agriculture were concerned only with disease eradication. But now, we have come into what we feel a veterinarian's full function should be: the prevention of disease among animals and also the prevention of cruelty to them. I should think any veterinarian who likes animals would be proud to work for the Animal and Plant Health Inspection Service—indirectly, we help millions of animals.

13.

"Loving animals is not enough to get you through veterinary school."

The great pleasure of a dog is that you may make a fool of yourself with him and not only will he not scold you, but he will make a fool of himself too.

—SAMUEL BUTLER

So far in this book, you have read stories about veterinarians who are already in practice. This chapter is about the life of a veterinary student.

Tom Herrforth is finishing up his second year at one of the large Eastern veterinary colleges. He lives with his wife near the university campus. Emily Herrforth is a nurse in the university hospital. The young couple feel their respective training in the health professions will enable them to see a bit of the world—there are many countries where their skills would be welcome.

While every veterinary school is different, and no two students' experiences are exactly the same, Tom's impressions might be meaningful to a young person hoping to enter veterinary school.

I've been an animal-lover all my life. I had many pets as a child and even raised huskies during my high school years.

Somehow I was sidetracked from my desire to be a veterinarian. I got a college degree in literature and worked for a couple of years in a business firm. Gradually I made up my mind that I had to try to be a vet, no matter what it took. The obstacles looked insurmountable, I can tell you.

I had to go to night school at a college with a good prevet program for the science courses I was lacking. When finally, to my infinite surprise, I made it into veterinary school, I was older than most of my fellow students. As in most veterinary schools, about half the student body came from the preveterinary classes of the same university as the vet school. The competition for admission to veterinary school starts even there, in the prevet training.

And so, in giving you advice, I can't stress too much that the competition is fierce. Not only must you be a top student, but more and more admissions committees, I hear, are looking for well-roundedness—aptitudes in the humanities, wide interests, a range of activities. I don't think my degree in literature hurt me; it may even have helped in some way.

Also, I had worked in as many animal-related jobs as I could. Working as a veterinarian assistant is ideal, of course, but just being a receptionist in a vet's office, or putting up fences or shoveling manure on a dairy farm will give you points. Any way you can demonstrate a real desire for the profession helps.

A love for animals is the main reason most of us want to become vets, I suppose. But I can tell you that loving animals sure isn't enough.

If you are not admitted to vet school the first time you try, you can apply again—how many times depends on the individual school. I heard of a guy who got into Penn on his seventh try, and the joke goes that they finally let him in because they couldn't stand his bothering them in the admissions office any more.

Because there are so few veterinary schools, people from states that don't have them have an additional problem. The admissions office of a college has to give preference to applicants from within the state. So some students go to veterinary schools abroad. That's a possibility to consider if you have to. I know of people who have gone to vet school in Italy, Mexico, and the Philippines. The Veterinary Medical Association of New York City, 9 Rockefeller Plaza, can send you a list of foreign veterinary schools. You will have to pass board exams in order to practice in the U.S., though, so it's important to pick a school whose standards are high enough to prepare you. Be sure to ask the veterinary associations about the standards and requirements of each foreign school.

I think most veterinary students, at least in American schools, have a very tense and fearful first year. At my school, if you fail one course, out you go. A grade below 60 is failing. But out of seventy-two people in my class, only one has failed so far; another three have left simply because they couldn't stand the pressure. You go to school from 9:00 to 5:00 five days a week and study every evening and all weekend.

So far in my first two years, everything has been rote learning. How well you do depends largely on your ability to memorize facts. Also, you will have to learn the terms, the jargon of the profession. That is maybe 1,000 words you never heard before. And some courses—organic chemistry, for one—seem to be pure exercises in memory; I can't imagine how I will ever apply them in my work. According to the seniors, it's not until later on in veterinary school that you synthesize what you have learned and begin to use it. Just remember, in the beginning you'll do very little creative thinking or reasoning.

My experience has been that the first exams in any course are extremely hard; subsequent ones get progressively easier. The professors seem to take you over the more difficult hurdles first.

I hope to become a small-animal practitioner and specialize in dogs. The body of veterinary knowledge is expanding greatly, and my impression is that more and more vets are planning to specialize in certain animals, or to practice certain medical specialties such as cardiology, ophthalmology, or orthopedics. A few students I know plan to do pure research.

A number of us will probably go into medical research, at a university or for a private company or for the government. One organization doing a great deal of interesting research is the Public Health Service, a branch of the U.S. Government. I met a guy who graduated last year who is now working for the U.S. Center for Disease Control, studying one of the important zoonoses—those are animal diseases that can be transmitted to humans. It is a fairly new area of study, because while some 150 such diseases have been identified, comparatively little is known about them. Unfortunately, in several areas of the world where certain zoonoses are prevalent, they have been poorly diagnosed and scantily reported. Now, a number of international health organizations are getting interested in them and exchanging information.

Food safety is another area where veterinarians are needed, both by the Public Health Service and the Department of Agriculture. This specialty is likely to be of increasing importance in feeding the world's people.

Another vet I know has joined the Armed Forces to work in the Air Force Military Dog Veterinary Service.

He says about 2,000 dogs a year "join" the Air Force—for scouting, guarding, research. He and other veterinarians working with these dogs not only screen the "applicants" but give them medical and dental treatment to keep them healthy. In another branch of the Air Force, veterinarians conduct studies with chimpanzees and other primates at the School of Aviation Medicine in an aerospace medical center. The military uses over 1,000 veterinarians and veterinary technicians.

One girl in my class, Barbara Newman, is a terrific horsewoman and wants to work with racehorses, either as a racetrack vet or at a thoroughbred farm. She met the manager and resident veterinarian of a thoroughbred farm who is in complete charge of several hundred valuable racehorses. He handles their nutrition, breeding, preventive medicine—everything. Barbara decided that sort of work was for her and is taking additional courses in horse breeding and management to increase her qualifications.

About 2,000 veterinarians serve on the faculties of veterinary schools, teaching students and often doing research. Since most veterinary colleges have a clinic and hospital available to the public, the professors also treat animals, large and small.

If the approximate numbers of vets in these specialties I've been telling you about seem small—2,000 in this, 1,000 in that—you have to remember that there are only about 30,000 veterinarians in the United States at present. This is one field where there is still a demand rather than a surplus. So many people of my generation have been trained for fields which are already overcrowded. Not so this profession.

One other thing I might mention about veterinary school. Be prepared to see a certain amount of callousness toward animals' pain and even death. This came as a shock to me—I was very idealistic and thought I would find real dedication to animals and their welfare. But many of the teachers seem amazingly insensitive to animal suffering and impart this attitude to the students. I guess it's the same in human medicine, and perhaps a certain amount of toughness is necessary. I'm not sentimental—I just expected simple kindness toward the animals we work with, but I haven't always seen it. I was somewhat disillusioned.

Nevertheless, even with the competition, the pressure, the drudgery, and the disappointments of veterinary school, I still feel it's worth it in order to become a veterinarian.

Good luck to you.

How to Apply to
Veterinary School

_In 1977_

There are twenty-one veterinary schools or colleges (universities call them one or the other) in the United States and three in Canada. All but two of the American veterinary schools are at publicly supported state universities and therefore give preference to applicants from their own state. Some states that don't have veterinary colleges at present are planning to open them in the near future, and some states are considering joining with others to establish veterinary schools together, sharing the cost and giving priority to their own residents who qualify academically. Some states with veterinary schools have an arrangement with neighboring states for admitting students from those states.

Because there is so much interest in veterinary medicine, and a need for veterinarians, applicants to veterinary schools far surpass the number that can be admitted. If you wish to become a veterinarian, you are going to face very tough competition. You may have heard how hard it is to get into medical school—that is nothing compared to the perseverance and high qualifications you'll need to be accepted into veterinary school. Over one-third of the students who apply to medical school make it; for veterinary school, the number ranges from one in five to one in fifteen, depending on the school.

The very best way to increase your chances is to be a top student in high school, especially in science subjects. Then go to a college with a good preveterinary curriculum, and make high grades there too. An early step in your planning should be to contact the college of veterinary medicine to which you plan to apply. Each college sets its own requirements for admission, so you must be sure to take the right preveterinary courses.

All veterinary schools require at least two years of college preveterinary study; over 40 percent of the students admitted, however, have had four or more years of college. You will have to do well on a number of entrance exams. In addition, work experience helps—especially summer or part-time employment with a veterinarian or in an animal hospital. Your health, student activities, experience with animals, and interests count too.

If you are refused at the first schools you apply to, it is not necessarily the end of the world—you can reapply later on.

Veterinary school itself is a four-year program—the first two years of which are virtually the same as the first two of medical school. You will graduate with a Doctor of Veterinary Medicine or Veterinary Medical Doctor degree (DVM or VMD). You then have to pass a tough state licensing exam before you can practice.

Most veterinary colleges have some scholarships, loans,

awards, or part-time jobs available to students who need them.

In the past, relatively few women applied to veterinary school, and the schools admitted only a token few. This situation has changed so dramatically that now a qualified woman applicant has as good a chance of being admitted to veterinary school as a man. At present, women make up slightly over 20 percent of the student body at veterinary schools. So many girls are applying now that some estimates claim they may constitute 40 percent in the near future.

Following is a list of the schools and colleges of veterinary medicine that are accredited by the American Veterinary Medical Association:

UNITED STATES

School of Veterinary Medicine
Auburn University
Auburn, Ala. 36830

School of Veterinary Medicine
Tuskegee Institute
Tuskegee, Ala. 36088

School of Veterinary Medicine
University of California
Davis, Calif. 95616

College of Veterinary Medicine
    and Biomedical Sciences
Colorado State University
Ft. Collins, Colo. 80521

College of Veterinary Medicine
University of Florida
Gainesville, Fla. 32601

College of Veterinary Medicine
University of Georgia
Athens, Ga. 30601

College of Veterinary Medicine
University of Illinois
Urbana, Ill. 61801

School of Veterinary Medicine
Purdue University
W. Lafayette, Ind. 47907

College of Veterinary Medicine
Iowa State University
Ames, Iowa 50010

College of Veterinary Medicine
Kansas State University
Manhattan, Kans. 66502

College of Veterinary Medicine
Louisiana State University
Baton Rouge, La. 70803

College of Veterinary Medicine
Michigan State University
E. Lansing, Mich. 48823

College of Veterinary Medicine
University of Minnesota
St. Paul, Minn. 55101

College of Veterinary Medicine
University of Missouri
Columbia, Mo. 65202

New York State College
  of Veterinary Medicine
Cornell University
Ithaca, N. Y. 14850

College of Veterinary Medicine
Ohio State University
Columbus, Ohio 43210

College of Veterinary Medicine
Oklahoma State University
Stillwater, Okla. 74074

School of Veterinary Medicine
University of Pennsylvania
Philadelphia, Pa. 19104

College of Veterinary Medicine
University of Tennessee
Knoxville, Tenn. 37901

College of Veterinary Medicine
Texas A & M University
College Station, Tex. 77843

College of Veterinary Medicine
Washington State University
Pullman, Wash. 99163

CANADA

Ontario Veterinary College
University of Guelph
Guelph, Ontario, Canada

École de Médecine Vétérinaire
Université de Montreal
St. Hyacinthe, Quebec, Canada

Western College of Veterinary Medicine
University of Saskatchewan
Saskatoon, Saskatchewan, Canada

Note: As this book went to press, two additional colleges of veterinary medicine have been slated to open. For information, write: Mississippi State University, Mississippi State, Miss. 39762, and Virginia Polytechnic Institute, Blacksburg, Va. 24061.

How to Become an Animal Technician or Technologist

Larry S., a college freshman, would like to become a veterinarian, but his academic record is not high enough for him to meet the requirements for admission to a veterinary school. Joan B., a high school senior, wants to work with animals in some capacity, but without the many years of college required to become a veterinarian. Bill M., also a high school senior, wants to become financially independent in semiprofessional work related to the sciences within two years of graduation.

All three of these young people, and others with similar reasons, might consider a type of training that would qualify them to work in the broader field of veterinary medicine without becoming veterinarians. They might become Animal Technicians or perhaps Animal Technologists.

These are two new careers that have developed because of both the shortage of veterinarians and the need for trained veterinary assistants. Animal Technicians or Technologists are veterinarians' assistants or veterinary research assistants with special training in subjects within the profession of veterinary medicine.

Animal Technology is a four-year college program during which you earn a Bachelor of Science degree. You would be trained in routine animal care, nutrition, and breeding and in the treatment and prevention of animal diseases. You would know about diagnostic procedures and surgical assisting, and you could do any form of clinical work with animals as long as you were supervised by a veterinarian. You might administer anesthesia or take X rays. You could not make diagnoses, or perform surgery, or prescribe medicine, but you could assist a veterinarian in doing these things.

Besides working as a veterinarian's assistant, you might, with the Bachelor of Science degree, work in an animal hospital, a research laboratory, a zoo or museum, or a wildlife preserve or for a food or drug company. You could also hold a supervisory position in any of a number of large organizations.

An Animal Technician is similar to a Technologist, but has been trained in a two-year college program that gives an associate degree. He or she might be an assistant to a veterinarian and perform such duties as: obtaining and recording information about patients; preparing patients, instruments, equipment, and medications for surgery; collecting laboratory specimens and performing some laboratory procedures; dressing wounds; assisting a veterinarian in diagnostic, medical, and surgical procedures.

Or, if you are an Animal Technician and work for a research laboratory, a zoo, an animal breeder, or a food or drug company, you might supervise animal care and feeding, perform laboratory procedures, keep records, maintain equipment, perhaps manage an animal hospital office.

Job opportunities for both the Animal Technician and the Technologist are good.

To qualify for admission to a school with an Animal Technician program, you need at least a high school diploma or equivalency certificate. A strong background in science subjects is very advantageous. Other considerations are aptitudes, work experience, and recommendations of your high school counselor and/or employers.

Here are some of the subjects you would be likely to take in a good Animal Technician program: chemistry, mathematics, microbiology, pharmacology, anatomy and physiology, animal diseases, animal management, animal behavior, animal nutrition, laboratory animal technology, technical reporting, economics, animal hospital procedures. You must also put in many hours working in a veterinary clinic for credit.

Because these veterinary-related careers are so new, there are still some problems associated with them—for example, training varies widely from school to school. Not all programs meet the same standards or have the same objectives. There are very few standard textbooks or uniform exams for Animal Technician subjects. The schools and programs vary so much that a veterinarian wishing to hire an Animal Technician does not really know how well an applicant has been trained or what his or her capabilities are. The laws that apply to Animal Technicians also need to be clarified and defined.

To solve these problems, the American Veterinary Medical Association has established basic standards that must be met by a school in order for the school's Animal Technician program to be accredited (that is, "approved"). If you complete an accredited program, it means that your school has taught you certain basic subjects according to certain standards.

In the list below of schools offering programs for Animal Technicians or Technologists, those that have been accredited by the AVMA are marked with a star (*). However, since the situation is changing constantly, you would do well to obtain the AVMA's most recent and complete list when you are ready to apply to college. Write: American Veterinary Medical Association, 930 N. Meacham Rd., Schaumburg, Illinois 60172.

COLLEGES OFFERING ANIMAL TECHNICIAN OR TECHNOLOGIST PROGRAMS

ARKANSAS

Department of Animal Sciences 2 years
University of Arkansas
Fayetteville, Ark. 72701

CALIFORNIA

*Los Angeles Pierce College 2 years
6201 Winnetka Ave.
Woodland Hills, Calif. 92101

Yuba College 2 years
Yuba Community College District Associate in Science
Maryville, Calif. 95901

*Consumnes River College 2 years
8401 Center Parkway Associate in Science
Sacramento, Calif. 95823

Veterinary Science Department
California State Polytechnic
  College
San Luis Obispo, Calif. 93401

4 years
Bachelor of Science
(Proposed)

San Francisco School for
  Health Professions
1550 California St.
San Francisco, Calif. 94109

2 years

COLORADO

*Colorado Mountain College
803 Colorado Ave.
Glenwood Springs, Colo. 81601

2 years
Associate in Science

*Bel-Rea Institute of Animal
  Technology
9870 East Alameda
Denver, Colo. 80231

2 years
Associate in Applied
  Science & State
  Certification

CONNECTICUT

Quinnipiac College
Mount Carmel Ave.
Hamden, Conn. 06518

4 years
Bachelor of Science

FLORIDA

Department of Animal Science
Institute of Food & Agriculture
  Sciences
University of Florida
Gainesville, Fla. 32601

4 years
Bachelor of Science

St. Petersburg Junior College Box 13489 St. Petersburg, Fla. 33733	2 years Associate in Science

GEORGIA

Abraham Baldwin Agriculture College Tifton, Ga. 31794	2 years

ILLINOIS

Parkland College 2400 W. Bradley Champaign, Ill. 61820	2 years

KANSAS

*Colby Community College 1255 South Range Colby, Kans. 67701	2 years Associate in Applied Science

KENTUCKY

Morehead State University Box 702 Morehead, Ky. 40351	2 years

LOUISIANA

Department of Agricultural Sciences Northwestern State University of Louisiana Natchitoches, La. 71457	2 years Associate in Science

MAINE

Department of Animal and Veterinary Sciences University of Maine Orono, Maine 04473	2 years Associate in Science

MASSACHUSETTS

Department of Veterinary and Animal Science Stockbridge School of Agriculture University of Massachusetts Amherst, Mass. 01001	2 years Associate Degree (Applied Science)

MICHIGAN

*College of Veterinary Medicine Michigan State University East Lansing, Mich. 48823	2 years Certificate

MINNESOTA

Medical Institute of Minnesota 2309 Nicollet Ave. Minneapolis, Minn. 54404	2 years Associate in Science

*University of Minnesota Waseca Technical College Waseca, Minn. 56093	2 years Associate in Science

MISSISSIPPI

Hinds Junior College Raymond, Miss. 39154	2 years Associate in Applied Science

MISSOURI

*Maple Woods Community College   2 years
2601 N. E. Barry Rd.
Kansas City, Mo. 64156

NEBRASKA

*School of Technical Agriculture   2 years
University of Nebraska   Associate in Techni-
Curtis, Neb. 69025   cal Agriculture in
Veterinary Tech-
nology

NEW JERSEY

Camden County College   2 years
P. O. Box 200   Associate in Applied
Blackwood, N. J. 08012   Science

NEW YORK

*Veterinary Science Technology   2 years
    Department   Associate in Applied
Agricultural and Technical College   Science
State University of New York
Delhi, N. Y. 13753

Biomedical Technology Depart-   2 years
    ment   Associate in Applied
Agricultural and Technical College   Science
State University of New York
Farmingdale, N. Y. 11735

College of Health Related   4 years
   Professions   Bachelor of Science
State University of New York
Downstate Medical Center
450 Clarkson Ave.
Brooklyn, N. Y. 11203

NORTH CAROLINA

*Central Carolina Technical   2 years
   Institute   Associate in Applied
Rt. 2, Box 55   Science
Sanford, N. C. 27330

OHIO

*Columbus Technical Institute   2 years
550 East Springs Street   Associate in Applied
Columbus, Ohio 43215   Science
(In cooperation with the Ohio
   State University College
   of Veterinary Medicine)

*Raymond Walters College   2 years
University of Cincinnati   Associate in Science
Cincinnati, Ohio 45221

OREGON

Portland Community College   2 years
Portland, Ore. 97219   Associate in Science

PENNSYLVANIA

Harcum Junior College
Bryn Mawr, Pa. 19010

2 years
Associate in Applied
Science

TENNESSEE

Columbia State Community
   College
Columbia, Tenn. 38401

2 years
Associate in Science

TEXAS

*Texas State Technical Institute
James Connally Campus
Waco, Tex. 76705

2 years

Range Animal Science Department
Sul Ross State University
Alpine, Tex. 78830

2 years

Biomedical Science Program
Department of Veterinary Public
   Health
College of Veterinary Medicine
Texas A & M University
College Station, Tex. 77843

4 years
Bachelor of Science

Frank Phillips College
Borger, Tex. 79007

2 years

VERMONT

Department of Animal Pathology
University of Vermont
Burlington, Vt. 05401

4 years
Bachelor of Science

VIRGINIA

Blue Ridge Community College   2 years
Box 80   Associate in Science
Weyers Cave, Va. 24486

WASHINGTON

Northwest College for Medical and   2 years
   Dental Assistants   Associate in Animal
1305 Seneca St.   Technology
Seattle, Wash. 98122

Department of Animal Sciences   4 years
Washington State University
Pullman, Wash. 99163

*Fort Steilacoom Community   2 years
   College   Associate in Animal
6010 Mount Tacoma Drive, S.W.   Technology
Tacoma, Wash. 98499

WISCONSIN

*Madison Area Technical College   2 years
211 North Carroll St.
Madison, Wis. 53703

WYOMING

Eastern Wyoming College   2 years
3200 West C St.
Torrington, Wyo. 82240

CANADA

ONTARIO

St. Lawrence College of Applied Arts and Technology Box 6000 Kingston, Ontario, Canada	3 years Diploma
Ontario Department of Agriculture and Food Centralia College of Agricultural Technology Huron Park, Ontario, Canada	2 years Diploma
St. Clair College of Applied Arts and Technology 2000 Talbot Rd. Windsor, Ontario, Canada	2 years Diploma

SASKATCHEWAN

Kelsey Institute of Applied Arts and Sciences Box 1520 Saskatoon, Saskatchewan, Canada	2 years

The History of
Veterinary Medicine

Let's say you are a young man or woman living in prehistoric times. Your tribe has domesticated several kinds of animals and established some sort of primitive agriculture. You have a wolflike animal, probably the ancestor of the modern dog, who hunts with you and helps guard the livestock you keep. One day this animal injures his leg. Because he is useful to you, and because you also feel a certain affinity toward him, you decide to treat his injury. You fashion a sort of splint out of a piece of bark and wrap it around the animal's leg with reeds and grasses to protect the leg until it heals.

Sound farfetched? Maybe. But this could have been the way veterinary medicine began. The cave paintings of early people show that they knew some basic principles of biology—for instance, they knew the location of an animal's heart and understood its importance. When human beings started to use some animals as hunting assistants and to domesticate others for food, milk, hides, work, and transportation, they probably also began to take an interest in the animals' health and well-being.

Thousands of years later, the people of certain civilizations incorporated animals into their religions. And since animals played significant roles, most likely some kind of care was given to them. But the chances are that animal medicine developed most rapidly in places where, because of climate or location, there was a high incidence of disease. For example, the fertile Nile River delta in East Africa is known to have been the birthplace of plagues that affected animals and human beings alike. Because this area was a big center of trade, diseases were quickly transmitted to other parts of the world. We can only guess at the sort of medical care given to the animals of the very earliest civilizations since there are no records detailing it. But we do know that the Code of Hammurabi, a set of laws proclaimed by that Babylonian king about 2,250 years B.C., includes several references to the practice of animal medicine. This means that it was already an actual professional service, subject to regulation by law.

It's interesting that the early Greeks, who were highly advanced in other fields, and especially in medicine, make little mention of veterinary medicine. Possibly the science existed, and we just haven't found records of it. But another reason for its absence in the Greeks' writings could be that the incidence of animal disease was relatively low in the arid, healthy climate of the Aegean lands. We do know that Aristotle, who was a notable biologist, performed dissections on animals and made accurate records of structural differences and similarities.

Ancient Chinese cultures also produced great medical works and had an advanced agriculture but left only a few records of veterinary work. Some treatises going back as far as 2,500 B.C. do exist on diseases of horses, camels, and buffalo, and records indicate that acupuncture was (as it still is) used in China in the treatment of animals. In Japan, it appears that farmers with sick livestock were able to obtain government aid, and that straw sandals were used to protect horses' hooves, but little else is known about the care of Japanese animals in ancient times.

There is, however, ample evidence that Korea had a well-developed veterinary field, headed by veterinary priests. These priests so impressed a member of the Imperial Court that he established a veterinary hospital in 598 A.D. And one record notes that special housing was provided for sick horses. By the eighth century, vets enjoyed good professional standing, and many were sent to China to study medicine. Killing or injuring an animal was a capital offense in seventeenth-century Korea, punishable with beheading.

During the Vedic period in India, which lasted from about 1,500 to 500 B.C., some outstanding work went on in veterinary medicine. The Hindu people regarded animals as kin to humans and treated them with enormous respect. Medicine was recognized as an art separate from religion, and this approach generated a scientific development free of sorcery and mystical hocus-pocus—which hasn't happened in many civilizations, either before or since! Unfortunately, not many Vedic doctrines were translated, but the few papers that we know of were remarkably advanced, and they influenced work in the field of science centuries later.

The first Indian veterinary hospital was established about 250 B.C. by King Asoka, a great humanitarian and friend of animals. Several others were founded during Asoka's reign, all government funded. Punishments for cruelty to animals were severe—imagine such a thing today—and owners were required by law to give an accounting of all illnesses or deaths among their animals. Other government policies guaranteed decent care to animals, and sanctuaries were provided for the sick and old. India led the world in veterinary care for hundreds of years.

In the Roman economy, which rested on slave power, animals had very low status. Animals that became useless were cruelly driven away. The incidence of plague was high in Rome, however, and the threat to the population finally created a need for veterinary medicine. In fact, the word *veterinarian* comes from the Latin *veterinarius*, which means "pertaining to cattle." In the first century A.D., a famous Roman agriculturist named Varro became concerned about the health of animals in relation to the health of people. Varro recognized contagion, and his ideas anticipated the germ theory of disease. These concepts were very advanced for a time when illness was generally believed to be a form of punishment inflicted by heavenly powers upon people who weren't reverent enough.

Despite a growth of medical knowledge among scholars, the general population inflicted barbaric forms of "treatment" on animals. The practice of "bleeding" (taking blood from a vein) was popular—it was believed to extract "bad blood" from the animal. The sicker the animal, the more it was bled, frequently from major veins like the jugular—the big one in the neck. Sometimes people would pour concoctions down the throats and even the nostrils of sick animals, a practice that surely hastened many to their death from drowning. During one anthrax epidemic, people poured enough of a deadly concoction down the throats and noses of their cows to kill off large numbers of animals that didn't even have symptoms of the disease.

The Roman Catholic Church of those days was opposed to veterinary science because it recognized the biological connection between human beings and animals, which challenged the Church's theory of the unique creation of mankind. Animals were considered to have no souls and therefore to be unworthy of serious attention. Any writings that questioned Church doctrine were destroyed. In 391 A.D., the huge library of the Byzantine Empire at the University of Alexandria was burned down by religious fanatics. Approximately 700,000 volumes were destroyed, including the medical doctrines of some of the most advanced thinkers of ancient times.

Despite the opposition of the Church, two significant works on veterinary medicine were published during this time; one of them, *Books of the Veterinary Art*, was actually written right under the nose of the Church. Its author, the Roman Vegetius Renatus, is sometimes referred to as "the father of veterinary medicine." Vegetius pointed out the need for a well-developed veterinary science and condemned the gruesome acts performed on animals in the name of medicine. The other work on veterinary science was a tenth-century Byzantine anthology called the *Hippiatrika* that included writings of 156 Greek and Byzantine authors. Many of the animal doctors whose writings appear in the *Hippiatrika* believed in natural rather than supernatural causes of disease. These books remain landmarks of their period, a time when scientific investigation was considered subversive.

The Renaissance period in Europe brought a rebirth of scientific thinking, and interest in the veterinary arts was revived. During the reign of Frederick II of Sicily, universities sprang up throughout Italy, and a medical school was established at Salerno. King Frederick even appointed a nobleman named Jordanus Ruffus as court veterinarian. With his high position and the support of the king, Jordanus did much to elevate the status of veterinary medicine; he also wrote books on the subject.

By the sixteenth century, some small veterinary schools had been founded in Spain. Veterinary literature was coming out of Spain, England, and France, but translations were scarce, and reliable information wasn't widely circulated. As a result, every animal owner became a self-appointed veterinarian. Many even wrote books filled with misconceptions and popular cures. Because the public was more apt to accept superstition than scientific fact, these homespun remedies were widely practiced. Such books held back the progress of veterinary medicine.

One exception was a book called *The Anatomy of the Horse*, written by an Italian lawyer named Carlo Ruini in 1598. Ruini's book contained accurate observations made from his extensive dissections of horses—a practice that was rarely used. It was illustrated with beautiful pictures of equine anatomy that are thought possibly to have been drawn by the great Renaissance artist Titian. Ruini suggested that blood circulates inside the body, although the famous English physician William Harvey is generally given credit for this discovery. Unfortunately, Ruini wasn't taken seriously, nor was his book widely circulated.

Due to technical improvements in the printing process by the end of the seventeenth century, books were more available to the general public. Yet the existing body of medical knowledge had very little effect on the treatment of animals—or humans. Surgery was performed on people by the local barber and on horses by the farrier, or blacksmith. Survival rates for surgery were very low. In the process of shoeing—something that should no more hurt a horse than a manicure hurts people—horses were sometimes crippled for life. Animals were still bled—in fact, cow doctors were called "cow leeches," and were even less respected than farriers. For the most part, farriers, cow leeches, and animal owners who attempted to treat their animals themselves were all more of a menace than a help.

Then, in 1713, the outbreak of a plague known as rinderpest called attention to the need for well-trained veterinary practitioners. This disease affects cattle mostly, but sheep, goats, and pigs are susceptible as well. In some areas of Europe, the people had sense enough to quarantine and slaughter infected animals to prevent the spread of the disease. Losses were nevertheless severe; in France, half of the cattle population was destroyed by plague during the eighteenth century.

Finally, in 1761, a famous French horseman named Charles Bourgelat established a medical school at Lyons devoted to research of animal diseases. This became the Royal Veterinary School; two years later, a branch hospital was opened at Alfort. These schools marked the recognition in modern times of veterinary medicine as a separate science and of the value and necessity of highly trained practitioners. The school at Lyons attracted students from all over Europe, many of whom were already physicians. In 1791 the Veterinary College of London was established, and by the end of the century, one or more veterinary schools existed in every major European country. These veterinary schools expanded their scope of study to include sheep and hogs as well as cows and horses. Small animals were eventually included too, partly because of repeated distemper epidemics in urban areas.

In America during the nineteenth century, the rapid growth of agriculture and its importance to our economy led to a demand for veterinary services. But the practitioners of the time were disreputable horse traders, motivated by financial profit. The fact that most horse traders did consider themselves veterinarians qualified to practice reflects the low standards of veterinary care. In 1847, there were only fifteen graduate vets in the entire country, all of whom had been trained in veterinary schools abroad.

The veterinary practice of eighteenth- and early nine-teenth-century America has been referred to ironically by one historian as "The Golden Age of Quackery." The atrocities performed on sick animals hastened thousands, perhaps millions, to their deaths in agony. Homespun remedies included forcing thin horses to drink sewage to fatten them, tearing out the soles of their feet for a disease called founder, driving cattle through bonfires to prevent plague, driving spikes in the heads of cattle to cure an imaginary disease called "hollow horn," and thrusting red-hot pokers into the rectums of animals as a remedy for a condition called bloat.

Some of the first people to show concern for the sorry state of the veterinary profession here were members of an organization called the Philadelphia Society for Promoting Agriculture. Early in the 1800s, articles began appearing in the society's publication, *Memoirs*, stressing the need for extensive research in animal diseases. *Memoirs* published what was really the first veterinary literature in America. The publication reported cases of disease and is the oldest record of animal plagues here. Many agricultural publications, which were widely read by farmers, began to run columns and articles on veterinary-related topics.

The books written by a veterinarian named George Dadd were also popular. The first, *Modern Horse Doctor*, was published in 1845; *American Cattle Doctor* appeared four years later. Despite their down-home sounding titles, these books embodied concepts that were scientifically advanced and condemned some of the widespread, barbaric practices like bleeding and pouring toxic concoctions down the throats (or nostrils) of sick animals. Dadd also urged that general anesthesia be used during surgery on animals, although unfortunately this wasn't practiced for another forty years.

The incidence of animal plagues—pleuropneumonia and rinderpest, for example—had never been as high on this continent as it was in Europe. So long as the density of the population was low, herds were so widely separated that disease didn't spread very rapidly. The lack of efficient transportation was another factor that prevented animal plagues. The diseases animals did have were related to their living conditions—unsanitary barnyards or pastures, which created an infection-prone environment. Also, when animals were malnourished because grass-crop yields were poor, their resistance to illness was lowered.

With the growth of populations and the improvement of transportation systems, however, the spread of disease became a problem. The knowledge of animal diseases that had accumulated in Europe could not always be applied in America. Although our livestock were largely European in origin, both the environment and the types of common parasites here were different and changed the nature of the European animal illnesses. And so American livestock were prey to diseases that weren't familiar to veterinarians trained abroad and weren't mentioned in contemporary textbooks.

The middle of the nineteenth century marked a turning point in the history of veterinary medicine in America. The increase in population brought about a rise in demand for dairy and meat products. Improved railroad networks and the use of refrigerated railroad cars encouraged the growth of this demand, and people began to be interested in improving the quality and developing new breeds of dairy and meat animals. At the same time, however, terrible plagues were threatening American livestock, and of course the afflicted animals were unfit for consumption. After the U.S. Department of Agriculture was founded in 1862, a movement was started to institute a well-organized veterinary department within it.

The same year, President Lincoln approved the Morrill Land Grant College Act, which appropriated public land to each state. Funds from the sale of these lands were to be used to further research and establish agriculture schools. Most schools at that time which had agriculture departments also offered courses in veterinary medicine or even had departments of veterinary science. In 1863, the U.S. Veterinary Medical Association was founded—the first such organization in the world.

Texas fever was one of the most dangerous diseases affecting American livestock in the nineteenth century. Veterinarians were stumped for some years because they couldn't discover its cause. Bitter regional controversies developed over Texas fever. In those days cattle of southern Texas and Mexico were driven or "trailed" across the Midwest to Eastern markets. The Texas cattle, which were Mexican and Spanish in origin, were able to make the journey successfully, but they left a path of death behind them. As they crossed the country, they would come in contact with other breeds of cows that were European in origin—and those cows would suddenly sicken and die. The farmers of the Midwest and the East were up in arms about the destruction of their stock by Texas fever, which they correctly guessed was transmitted by the Southwestern cattle, who weren't affected by it. The farmers waged a battle to prevent trailing, and even threatened to shoot any Texas cattle that attempted to come through their state.

To deal with problems of this nature, the Bureau of Animal Industry was created within the Department of Agriculture by an act of Congress in 1884. Its purpose was to prevent the importation of diseased animals into the United States and to suppress and exterminate diseases occurring among native livestock. This act is also known as the Hatch Act, after a Missouri congressman named William Hatch, who was largely responsible for it.

More bitter argument went on within the BAI about Texas fever. Finally, in 1904, after twenty-five years of research, the mystery was solved. The disease was found to be carried by a certain tick native to Mexico and the Southwestern United States. Local cattle were immune to the disease the tick carried, but other breeds weren't.

The discovery of the source of Texas fever established an important medical fact: diseases could be transmitted by insects. This led to the discovery that malaria and yellow fever were carried by mosquitoes.

Texas fever wasn't the only animal disease that was eliminated by the Bureau of Animal Industry. Pleuro-pneumonia, the cattle sickness that had caused many deaths among children who drank milk from infected cows, was effectively wiped out. Hog cholera, the first native American plague, had caused millions of dollars' worth of losses until the BAI was successful in eradicating it in 1890. More recently, in the late 1940s, work and research were carried out in a joint effort by the BAI and Mexican veterinarians to combat foot-and-mouth disease, which had caused severe losses in Mexico and was beginning to invade this country.

Other contributions of Congressman Hatch's were the Hatch Act of 1887, which allocated federal funds to state agricultural colleges for research, including veterinary research, and the Meat Inspection Act of 1890, which made American meat safe to eat.

The twentieth century brought social changes that had an important impact on the veterinary profession. The shift from horsepower to machine power for agriculture and industry caused a great decline in the economic value of the horse. But as dependence on the horse declined, another kind of dependence rose—Americans' need for meat in their diets. The public was aware that the veterinary profession had become indispensable to the raising of healthy animals for meat. Unfortunately, the cost of a veterinary education had increased, and the private veterinary schools which had cropped up in the 1800s began to go under—one reason for the shortage of veterinarians that still exists today. At the same time, interest in small animals as pets increased, creating a demand for small-animal practitioners and leading to the foundation of many animal hospitals. Veterinary researchers began to collaborate and share information with medical researchers in combating diseases that are similar in animals and humans and diseases that are communicable between them. During World War II, the work of veterinarians in the military created the Army Veterinary Corps.

The BAI was replaced by the Agricultural Research Service and then in 1971 became the Veterinary Services division of the Animal and Plant Health Inspection Service, a part of the Department of Agriculture. It is still carrying on its work of protecting American animals from native and imported diseases. Two important victories in recent years were the eradication of Venezuelan equine encephalomyelitis (horse sleeping sickness) and exotic Newcastle disease, the deadly sickness of birds and poultry.

Veterinarians working for federal, state, and city governments today are involved in public health, experimental medicine, space medicine, drug research, meat and poultry inspection, studies of food products, and research on zoonoses—the diseases that are transmitted from animals to human beings.

Today's veterinarian, whether in private practice, research, teaching, public health, regulatory medicine, or the military, is engaged in varied and sophisticated work that is important to the well-being of the people of this country as well as to that of our animals. Unaware of the wide range of work that veterinarians do, and of the high standards of the profession, the public in general still tends to think of veterinarians mainly as animal doctors who treat pets. Nevertheless, informed scientists and other professionals consider the veterinarian today of equal standing —a long, long way from the "horse doctor" of centuries past. Perhaps the art will eventually come full circle to the prestige it enjoyed in ancient India or Korea.